the HEALING
POWER of FOOD

CHERYL REID

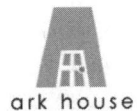

© Ark House Press

Ark House Press
PO Box 163
North Sydney, NSW, 2059
Telephone: (02) 8437 3541; Facsimile (02) 9999 2053
International: +612 8437 3541; Facsimile +612 9999 2053

All rights reserved. No part of this publication may be reproduced, stored in a retrieval system or transmitted in any form or by any means electronic, mechanical, photocopying, recording or otherwise without the prior written permission of the publisher. Short extracts maybe used for review purposes.

© Cheryl Reid 2005

Cataloguing in Publication Data:

Reid, Cheryl.
The healing power of food

Includes index.
ISBN 0 9752044 8 3.

1. Nutrition. 2. Health. 3. Cookery (Natural foods). I. Title.

613.2

Printed by: Southwood Press
Cover design by: Nicole Danswan

Disclaimer
No responsibility is accepted by the author or publisher for health remedies or advice expressed herein. The reader should always seek medical advice from qualified health professionals.

We would like to thank Gary Martin, naturopath, and the team at Living Valley Springs for awakening us to the real causes of disease and to the healing power of food.

We acknowledge Phillip Day, author and health reporter, for his investigation into the truth surrounding lifestyle diseases, thereby empowering people to take control of their own health and healing.

Samuel Epstein, chairman of the Cancer Prevention Coalition, has also been a source of vital information, bringing before the public the environmental causes of cancer and its prevention.

Introduction

This book is not a book for the conservative, the crowd-follower, the faint-hearted, or the unadventurous. It is not a book for those who would prefer the easy way out, or for those who are unprepared to rethink their eating habits.

It is about taking a serious, scientific look at the food of Western Society, and being willing to exchange bad habits for good. Based on life experience, this book contains a prescription for healing. The basic principle is simple: eliminate foods that are detrimental to health and replace them with foods that heal. The concept is older than Hippocrates, who wrote, "Let food be your medicine."

This book is not for those who want to 'go on a diet' for a while. It is about changing your lifestyle. If you are concerned for your health and want to maintain fitness into old age, then take a serious look at the evidence. Take the courage to eat differently…differently to the way you have eaten in the past, differently to the way our society eats and differently to the way the advertising media demand you should eat. Take a fresh look at food and discover its healing power.

CONTENTS

Part A: Food for Thought..7

1. The problem with food..9

2. Understanding the food we eat.....................................13

3. The best foods to eat..35

4. Practical aspects of eating for health............................39

5. Coping with cancer...51

6. Do we really know the cause of cancer?.......................57

7. Diet for cancer patients...67

8. Food supplements for everyone....................................85

9. Deadly lifestyle diseases...93

10. Made to be healthy...105

Part B: Recipes...114

FOREWORD
Gary Martin, Naturopath, Living Valley Springs

Cheryl Reid has aggressively researched food, nutrition and general lifestyle for many years, firstly to save her husband's life and then to share her knowledge with a world that is experiencing a rapid decline in well-being and longevity.

In 1997, Cheryl's husband Paul was diagnosed with terminal cancer. As a family they explored the options. Conventional Medicine offered little hope of survival. Orthomolecular medicine, which is the art of making one's food one's medicine, offered a lot more. Under the Orthomolecular model, in the case of sickness, the cause should be ascertained first. Conditions that do not promote health should be changed and wrong habits corrected. Then nature is to be assisted in her efforts to expel impurities and to re-establish right conditions in the system.

Paul and Cheryl reviewed their lives. Lifestyle habits, spinal and dental health, exposure to toxins and poor nutrition were all addressed. Paul spent ten days at the Living Valley Springs Health Retreat in Queensland. He also underwent dental revision, and then with Cheryl's help, established a new and exciting eating program designed to provide optimum nutrition with minimum exposure to toxins.

Cheryl cleaned out her cupboards replacing devitalised foods with fresh fruit and vegetables, whole grains, legumes, nuts, seeds and herbs. She studied hard as if her husband's life depended on it - and it did! She learned how to supply the body with a proper balance of protein, fats, carbohydrates, minerals and enzymes. Then Cheryl developed recipes to enhance the flavor and presentation of her meals.

Within eighteen months, Paul was given a clean bill of health, and has since enjoyed a healthy and happy cancer-free state. During that time Cheryl has influenced the lives of thousands of other victims who had little hope of long-term survival. Her first book, 'Food For Life' was published in 1998 and has helped many people to realise that we all need to take responsibility for our own health. Cheryl cares about you and your children. In this book she has provided a simple and easy plan so that you too can make your food your medicine.

Gary Martin ND
Founder and Director of Living Valley Springs Health Retreat
www.lvs.com.au

part A:
FOOD for THOUGHT

chapter one

The PROBLEM with FOOD

First the bad news...

No longer can we depend on supermarkets and restaurants for all our nutritional needs. Much of the food we buy lacks the essential vitamins and minerals we need for a healthy body. This is partly due to the depletion of vitamins and minerals in our soils, and food processing. Our food not only lacks the goodness that it once had, but may also contain toxic chemicals, preservatives, artificial colourings and flavourings and the list goes on.

Now the good news...

An understanding of good nutritional principles and a genuine desire to put them into practice can set your family on the road to good health. A healthy immune system is essential in a world where viruses are rampant, despite attempts by medical science to eliminate them. It is the responsibility of parents to set the example for their children, by eating the right food. This includes making the correct choices when buying and cooking food. It is also the responsibility of parents to have a correct understanding of nutrition and to educate their children accordingly.

The amount of junk food children consume these days is phenomenal. The media bombards us with compelling images of junk food and false information about nutrition. We need to get our children on our side and help them to understand the motives of the hidden persuaders. Children must understand that the media is trying to deceive them.

It was not until my husband, Paul, was diagnosed with terminal cancer that I started to understand the importance of food. I always thought we ate a healthy diet. I used a decoder, which indicated the safe and unsafe product numbers for food additives. We ate very little junk food, consumed only a little refined sugar and drank tea in moderation. However, as we looked into the cause of cancer we realised that our diet needed improving.

For Paul, a change of diet was a matter of life or death, and he depended on me to help him make that change. Had it not been for a life-threatening illness we would not have investigated diet to such a degree. I now realise that the knowledge we have gained by thoroughly researching the food issue, is knowledge that is vital for every family, whether they are faced with a life-threatening illness or not. The effects of bad eating habits may not show up for years to come. This is important to keep in mind with children. Children may appear to be perfectly healthy, existing quite happily on a mixed diet of healthy food and junk food. However, we do not know what problems will occur later in life due to accumulated toxins. Allergies and cancer are just two.

"But surely it is not possible to get children completely off junk food," you may say. My own children responded in a way that I wouldn't have believed possible. They not only liked the change of diet, but also even refused junk food of their own accord. I made a policy never to be a dictator when it came to abstaining from certain foods. This of course only applied when we were eating out, because at home there was no junk food to be found. I didn't say, "You can't have this and you can't have that!" I let them make their own decisions. To my amazement they always made the healthy choices.

Now this is not an automatic response. It actually comes from a lot of hard work. Education about food should be part of a child's total education, and the home is the best place for it. We took advantage of every opportunity to explain why we do or do not eat certain foods. We explained the problems with sugar, food additives, fast foods and fried foods. We explained the healing and disease-fighting properties of fresh fruit and vegetables. Food is actually an easy thing to talk about with children because we eat three times a day. You do not need to sit them down and say, "Now kids, we are going to have a lesson on food!" You just casually say as they are eating their broccoli, "Do you know why this broccoli is so important?"

You cannot expect children to change overnight. It is a gradual process of setting the example and educating them. It is working with them and encouraging them to change, rather than dictating. They must learn to make their own decisions, or they will revert to their old ways when you are out of sight! Of course consistency is another important factor. You can't say, "Well today we will eat junk food and tomorrow we will make up for it by eating broccoli." Healthy eating must be a lifestyle.

"Good news?" you might say. "Do I have to eat healthy food for the rest of my life?" Eating healthy food and actually enjoying it is an acquired process. You may not be able to change immediately, but at least work towards it. As time goes by, with the right mental attitude, you will find that you really enjoy healthy eating and actually dislike the junk food that you used to eat.

I hope that you will find many satisfying and delicious recipes in this book. You will also come to appreciate the delicious taste of the food that God's creation has provided for us. We have been provided with a huge variety of fruits, vegetables, grains, nuts and seeds, which have wonderful flavours. Too often we disguise that flavour with salt, sugar or sauce, so that we do not really appreciate the subtle flavours of food in its natural form.

Bon appetit!

Five basic principles for good nutrition

1. Eat mostly plant foods.
2. Minimise commercially processed foods.
3. Don't eat or drink anything that will have a harmful effect on your body, (short-term OR long-term).
4. Don't eat in between meals but drink plenty of liquid instead. (Make sure it's healthy liquid. Water is best.)
5. Don't over eat...even healthy food...and don't eat a large meal before going to bed. The digestive system works more slowly while you are asleep. Going to bed with undigested food in your stomach allows toxins to build up.

chapter two

UNDERSTANDING the FOOD we EAT

In order to make the right choices we need to understand the food we eat. Until recently there has been little research in the area of nutritional science. As research advances, new findings emerge. Many nutritional ideas from the past are now thought to be incorrect. How do we know where to find the right advice? Don't obtain nutritional information from the media. It can be slanted, geared to make you buy the product at any cost. You will hear many conflicting ideas about nutrition. Some people say, "If there's so much conflicting advice, then why bother listening to any of it. Why not just eat what you like?"

It is important that you don't throw the baby out with the bath water. Search for truth and you will find it. There is much reliable scientific research around. There are many sound books in health shops, but there are also many books that are not scientifically based. Be discerning. Read as much information as you can find. You will soon find a consistency of truth among the best sources of information. As well as books, there are some good Internet sources, such as Phillip Day's e-club bulletin, available through www.credence.org.

Not everyone responds to the same diet. You need to find out the requirements of your body. Underweight people will have different requirements to overweight people.

Growing children have different requirements to full-grown adults. However there are some basic common factors that should be taken into consideration for all diets. A predominance of vegetables, fruits, nuts, seeds and grains in their natural form is the healthiest way to go.

Fruit and vegetables

These are essential for our daily intake of vitamins and minerals. In their raw form, plant chemicals present in fruit and vegetables will protect us from free radical damage in our cells. These plant chemicals are called antioxidants.

Everyone is susceptible to free radical damage. Free radicals are generated by our environment - from air, water, pollutants, sunlight, radiation, drugs, pesticides, chemicals, fried foods, alcohol and tobacco smoke. Free radicals are also produced as the natural by-products of oxygen metabolism, or simply breathing. Stress further increases their production.

Free radicals are unpaired oxygen electrons. These unpaired electrons attempt to stabilise themselves by stealing another oxygen molecule from a healthy cell and that cell dies. This sets off a chain reaction that is extremely destructive to cell metabolism. Free radical damage contributes heavily to the two biggest killers – heart disease and cancer.*1*

Free radical damage increases in a person's body with age. We all generate free radicals, but the problem arises when free radicals get out of control. Years ago, our foods contained enough vitamins and minerals to keep free radicals under control. The substances responsible for doing this task are called antioxidants. Examples of antioxidants are vitamins A, C and E, present in fruit and vegetables that have been grown in nutrient-rich soils, picked when ripe and eaten fresh. However today, our soils are depleted of minerals, and so is much of our food. Most fruit is picked early and artificially ripened. It is placed in storage, transported and marketed, and finally reaches the consumer devoid of antioxidants. Vegetables also lack vitamins and minerals.

The solution lies in eating fresh, organic, fruit and vegetables. Cruciferous vegetables in particular have good cancer-fighting properties. These include cabbage, broccoli, cauliflower, asparagus, and Brussels sprouts. Dark red grapes, onions and garlic are another source of excellent anti-oxidants. Grape seed extract and extract of white pine bark, available in supplement form, are even more powerful.

Growing your own fruits and vegetables is a good idea, but time consuming. If you haven't the time or space, herbs, particularly Italian parsley, can be grown in pots. Parsley is a wonderful source of iron. It can be picked fresh as you need it, and added to salads.

The healing power of living plants lies in more than their vitamins and minerals alone. Plants manufacture hundreds, perhaps thousands, of phytochemicals, (plant chemicals). These include living enzymes and special carbohydrates, called polysaccharides. Nutrients in whole plant foods complement each other in the hundreds of chemical reactions that body cells must process for optimum health, as well as providing the fuel for cell-to-cell communication. Research shows that many of the phytochemicals have anticarcinogenic properties, as well as providing protection against other degenerative diseases. These plant chemicals help us fight the viruses and diseases we come into contact with from day to day, and help us build a healthy immune system. 2

Cooking food can destroy living enzymes, as well as many vitamins, so eating raw fruit and vegetables is a distinct advantage. Always start lunch and dinner with raw vegetables, and start breakfast with raw fruit. This stimulates the digestive juices, and you will absorb far more nutrients that way. Having eaten a salad, you can then eat the cooked component of the meal. For vegetables like root vegetables, which need cooking, it is best to steam rather than boil, or bake without oil. Microwaves ovens and aluminium cookware should be avoided at all costs! *(See Chapter 7 for details on the problem with microwaves.)*

Whole grains

Wheat is not the best grain. Our modern wheat is a hybrid, and lacks some of the vitamins of the older variety, spelt. Spelt is far superior in nutritional value and contains some vitamin B17. Most wheat flour is contaminated with pesticides and moulds. People with allergies and candida should avoid wheat, and for the most of us, we are better off choosing other grains.

There are some good alternatives to wheat, including brown rice, barley, buckwheat, millet, quinoa and oats. Buckwheat and quinoa are not actually grains, and can usually be tolerated by people who have a problem with grains. Both are highly nutritious. Many grains other than wheat are also available as flour. Oats, especially whole oats, are also a good option. Commercially processed breakfast cereals are high in salt and most are high in sugar. The list of added vitamins sounds impressive but they are only added to replace some of those taken out in processing. These fortified vitamins are not even in an absorbable form.

Whole grains can be a good source of protein, fibre and B vitamins while being low in fat. Refined grains such as white rice have little food value. Refined white flour has nutrients removed and contains bleach. White flour also causes food to pass slowly through the body, a contributor to bowel cancer. [3]

Whole grains should be chewed, ground or cracked in order to obtain nutritional value. Multi-grain bread should therefore be avoided, unless the grains are ground or cracked. Hard whole-wheat grains pass through the body undigested, leaching vitamins and minerals from the body as they pass through.

Nuts and seeds

Nuts and seeds are important sources of minerals. They are particularly high in potassium, iron and phosphorus, which work together with the B vitamins. Many nuts and seeds are high in calcium. Two good sources are hazelnuts and sesame seeds. Almonds, brazil nuts, pine kernels and pistachio nuts are high in the B vitamins. Cashews contain vitamin C and sunflower seeds contain vitamins D and E. Nuts and seeds can be sprinkled on hot dishes such as stir-fried vegetables, sprinkled onto a breakfast fruit salad, combined in a crumble topping on stewed fruit, and provide a principle ingredient in home-made muesli or muesli slice. They can also be taken as snack food on a picnic or in a school lunch.

Nuts and seeds are high in protein as well as oil. It is much better to consume oil in its natural form rather than in a processed form. Nut spreads make a good substitute for butter and margarine. For people who are intolerant to nuts, sunflower seeds can be used as a substitute in recipes requiring nuts. Tahini, made from sesame seeds, is another nutritious spread.

Peanuts must not be categorised as nuts. They are actually a legume, and should be avoided because they are susceptible to growing a potentially carcinogenic mould. The nut spreads such as almond or hazelnut spread, available from health shops, are a good substitute for peanut butter.

Fats and oils

Fats and oils are an essential part of good nutrition, and are particularly important for growing children. The best fats and oils are those present in their natural state, in fruit, vegetables, nuts, seeds, coconuts, free-range eggs and mercury-free fish oil. Eggs, fish oils and maybe a little organic butter occasionally can be beneficial because they provide us with the fat-soluble vitamins A, D, E and K.

Saturated fats from meat and dairy products should be kept to a minimum. Meat and dairy fats today will contain high pesticide residue, since environmental pesticides accumulate in the fatty tissues of the animal. Many people try to avoid animal fat by trimming their meat. However this is not the complete answer. Red meat and pork contain fat even when there is no visible fat.

Processed vegetable oils cause a lot of trouble. These are present in margarine, cooking oil and processed baked foods. Cooking oils, and particularly margarine, become potentially carcinogenic during the manufacturing process if they are exposed to light and heat. These oils, called trans-fats, or polyunsaturated oils, can break and enter arterial walls. They rob us of nutrients and cause free radical damage and thus weaken arterial walls leading to heart disease. Canola oil is especially harmful as it creates a vitamin E deficiency. It may also cause heart lesions, immune deficiency, ageing and obesity. [4]

It is better to avoid cooking with oil, but if you do need to use a little oil for certain recipes, then cold-pressed olive oil can withstand heating without becoming carcinogenic. The best cold-pressed olive oils are sold in light-proof containers, and should be kept in the dark after opening. Oils should never be reheated. We must remember that using even the best vegetable oil lavishly, will create an imbalance that is never found in nature.

For good nutrition we should not avoid fat completely, but try to find the right type of fat in the right quantities. Cholesterol, which is often thought to be harmful, plays an important role in the diet. For example, a considerable percentage of our brain is composed of cholesterol. [5]

Some saturated fat in the diet, in the form of cold-extracted organic coconut oil can be beneficial. Coconut oil protects tropical populations from bacteria and fungus. It is extremely stable and can be left for a long time without developing rancidity. It is antiviral and provides protection for the brain. [6]

The two fats, omega-3 and omega-6, commonly known as essential fatty acids, are excellent for our health, particularly when taken together in the same quantities. Omega-3 is found primarily in fish oil. Studies conclude that mercury-free fish oil helps prevent heart disease, cancer, depression, diabetes, memory-loss, increases energy and resistance to colds and flu. Since most fish today have high levels of mercury contamination, it is very important to choose a high quality fish oil that has been independently lab-tested and found to be free of mercury and other toxins.

Ground flaxseed, or linseed, is a source of both omega-3 and omega-6. To obtain the nutrients they should be ground in a coffee grinder or nut grinder immediately before consuming. The actual seeds are preferable to flaxseed oil, which runs the danger of rancidity.

Plant foods containing omega-6 oils include olive oil, evening primrose seeds, avocado, borage, psillium seeds, pumpkin seeds or pepitas, sesame seeds, sunflower seeds and nuts. Obtaining oils from food in its natural form is the best way of taking the oils we need. Plant oils are best taken in the form of nuts, seeds and the vegetables themselves, rather than processed vegetable oils. 7

Meat and fish

Due to modern farming methods, animal protein may be high in chemical residue, antibiotics and growth hormones. Fish may contain toxic chemicals and heavy metals such as mercury and lead. Shark and other large fish in particular run a high risk of containing heavy metals. This is because large fish eat many smaller contaminated fish, accumulating heavy metals over time. Small fish, caught closer to the shore, collect industrial waste and can be equally toxic. Probably the only fish reasonably safe to eat are small deep-sea fish (sardines), or non-farmed (wild) salmon. 8

The number of viruses and diseases affecting animals is increasing. Unfortunately some of these can be transferred to humans. There are more than 200 known communicable diseases in animals, and about one-half of these are infectious to man. Research at William Angliss College, Australia, shows that all meat carries a large number of different bacteria. Undercooked meat can contain up to ten types of disease-causing bacteria that are not found in meat that is well-done. Australia's first recorded outbreak of the potentially fatal disease, toxoplasmosis, has been linked to the eating of rare kangaroo meat. Most meat picks up dangerous bacteria during the slaughtering and butchering process due to exposure to air, contaminated knives and machinery. One of the most dangerous types of bacteria found in meat is salmonella, which causes diarrhea and cramps, and can cause serious food poisoning. Another is escherichia, which causes internal bleeding and pneumonia. Minced meat carries the most risk, especially when used in hamburgers. This is because contaminated surface meat, being mixed through the burger, cannot be cooked to the high temperature required to kill bacteria. Related studies from Iowa College of Medicine, U.S.A., show that there is a link between the eating of hamburgers and cancer. Carcinogens formed by burnt beef have been named as a possible cause as well as poor quality beef. 9

It is important to thaw meat in the refrigerator and not on the bench top, as bacteria will multiply in meat that has been left unrefrigerated for a time. When using a knife to prepare meat, it is important that the knife does not touch cooked meats or other foods. Otherwise bacteria can be transferred.

The chicken industry is extremely affected by disease-causing bacteria. If it weren't for antibiotics in the stock feed, almost all chickens would be affected by the contagious virus, leucosis. It is thought that this virus may be able to be transferred to humans as leukemia. Eggs are susceptible to the virus too, so free-range eggs are the safest because the hens are less confined and therefore less susceptible to disease. Some free-range poultry farmers, although not using pharmaceutical antibiotics, still give their hens a type of antibiotic in the form of mouldy bread. Free-range eggs do not cause high cholesterol, whereas eggs from battery hens do.

The practice of feeding antibiotics to livestock has its problems. When human beings ingest the antibiotics stored in the meat, a resistance to antibiotics builds up in our bodies, and we may find that they won't work for us at times when we really need them.

Growth hormones also present a problem. Battery chickens are fed hormones while free-range chickens are not. Children who consume large amounts of meat containing growth hormones can undergo premature development.

Meats containing nitrate and nitrites are most dangerous. Nitrate is a colour fixative used in most preserved meats such as bacon, ham, metwurst sausage and hot dogs. In large amounts nitrate can result in respiratory failure. Nitrites are colour fixatives and preservatives, also used in processed meats. A study in Los Angeles County conducted between 1980 and 1987 found that children who consumed more than 12 hot dogs a month had nine times the normal risk of developing childhood leukemia. Children and infants were found to have a higher rate of brain tumours if their mothers consumed one or more hot dogs per week during pregnancy. Children who consumed hamburgers once per week were found to be at greater risk of lymphocytic leukemia.

Infinitesimal amounts of nitrites have caused cancers in tests on mice. *10*

Including too much meat in the diet can place undue stress on the digestive system. Red meat in particular, takes a long time to digest, and is also responsible for an acidic system. A highly acidic system, acquired by eating a predominance of animal protein, is a recipe for cancer. Traditionally, western society has believed that we need to eat a lot of meat for protein. Hence the daily 'meat and three veggies'.

Nutritional science has now discovered that we don't need nearly so much protein. In fact we can get all the protein we need from a good balance of fruit, vegetables, grains, pulses, nuts and seeds. In our concern for not getting enough protein, we end up getting too much. Because the body does not store excess protein, the waste products thrown off by the metabolism of excess protein put a strain on the liver and kidneys. Other effects of too much protein are early maturing, premature aging and degenerative diseases.

Meat does have the advantage of being high in iron, but iron can also be obtained from plant foods. Plant foods that are high in iron are whole grains, beetroot, parsley, sunflower seeds, pumpkin seeds and many green vegetables. A plant-based colloidal mineral supplement will ensure that you maintain the correct iron balance. Vitamin B12 and vitamin C as part of your supplementation program will help in the absorption of iron.

Vitamin B12 does not have to be obtained from meat. It can be obtained from eggs. For people on a total plant food diet, it is essential to take a supplement that contains vitamin B12 in order to maintain adequate iron levels.

Dairy products

Regular milk fat contains hormones, antibiotics and pesticides. Dairy milk is a major cause of allergies. Dairy foods are promoted for their calcium content, and yet the high protein content of milk causes minerals to be leached out of the bones. This is because too much protein causes acidity. The body then tries to neutralise the acidity, by drawing calcium out of the bones. Taking in too much calcium through dairy products can therefore increase the risk of calcium loss and osteoporosis.[11] Osteoporosis is also caused by hormonal imbalance *(See chapter 9)*.[12]

Fruit and vegetables are a better source of calcium than dairy products. Green beans and oranges are both quite high in calcium. With a lower protein intake, calcium needs fall correspondingly. People who eat lentils, dried peas and beans for their protein, in preference to meat and dairy products, receive adequate amounts of calcium. Women in third-world countries, with lower intake of protein, do not suffer from osteoporosis, despite giving birth to more children and nursing them.

Dairy milk not only has more protein than human milk, but it has a different kind that works well for cows and not for human beings. It is called 'casein' and causes calcium leaching. The enzyme lactose, present in dairy milk, requires breaking down by another enzyme, lactase. Humans do not have this enzyme, so the lactose goes straight to the bowel undigested. There, the lactose allows yeast to thrive, contributing to candida. Organic yoghurt is somewhat better, having the advantage of good bacteria that improves the digestibility.

Homogenisation of milk increases the availability of saturated fat to the cells because the fat particles are so tiny that the body can take them up more readily. This contributes to weight gain and heart disease.

Conventional cheeses, (e.g. cheddar), are higher in fat than cocktail sausages, and although lower in sodium, still well above the dietary guidelines set down by The Australian Food Report. It is interesting to notice that when Australians reduced their intake of red meat, their cheese intake increased. Vegetarians who just substitute cheese for meat have no health advantages over meat eaters. [13]

Eggs

Free-range eggs are good food value and do not pose a high cholesterol problem. Free-range chickens are less likely to suffer from the diseases of battery hens, and therefore their eggs will be safer. Eggs help us to eliminate heavy metals from the body.

Sugar

The simple sugars, glucose, dextrose, fructose and grape sugar, as they come in their natural states in fruits and plants, are excellent fuels for cells to use in producing energy and heat. However sucrose is a refined table sugar composed of one molecule each of fructose and glucose and is difficult for the body to break down. The process of breaking down sucrose into simple sugars places strain on the body's digestive system. The immune system is also weakened as the body puts energy into breaking down the sugar molecules. The body's store of vitamins and minerals are depleted as a result. Eating sugar creates a mineral deficit! Minerals, the catalysts for chemical reactions within the body, are absolutely essential and will be severely compromised by the eating of sugar.

All forms of processed sugar, whether in the form of white, brown or raw sugar, are bad for us, and highly addictive. The vitamins, minerals and other nutrients naturally occurring in raw sugar cane, are not present in processed sugar. Sugar produces an acidic body-system, and can lead to osteoporosis, diabetes, hypoglycemia, hyperactivity and retardation of brain development in children, and of course, tooth decay. [14]

Naturally occurring fruit sugars can be purchased as fruit concentrates. Honey and molasses are also good choices. However, the free use of sugar in any form will put strain on the digestive system. Fresh fruits and vegetables, together with whole grains and legumes are the best sources of fuel for body cells. [15]

Many people think that processed cane sugar is a good source of energy, but it actually only gives us a temporary boost, after which our energy level is lowered due to the hard work our body undergoes in breaking down the complex carbohydrates.

When we assess the sugar content of our diet, we need to be aware of the amount of refined cane sugar that is added to processed foods. We may not sprinkle sugar on our cereal or take it in our beverages, but how much do we eat in the form of tomato sauce, tinned foods, bread and other processed foods?

Salt

It is true that our body needs salt, but not refined table salt. Sodium chloride, (table salt), has been refined to a state that is useful only for flavour, and in the refining process has become toxic. Toxic ingredients are also added to give the salt its free-flowing nature. One side-effect is high blood-pressure and possibly cancer. There is one type of salt that is hand-harvested from the sea in such a way that it maintains the valuable sea minerals without toxicity. This is called 'macrobiotic sea salt' or 'Celtic salt' and is available from health shops. It is wet and grey looking, and not white like refined sea salt. When buying sea salt, make sure that it is the unrefined type, and not just white sea salt. Due to its rich variety of vital minerals, unrefined sea salt has healing properties. *16*

Vegetables contain salt in a perfectly natural and healthy form. In assessing your salt intake, you need to consider the three ways in which salt can be consumed. Firstly, the salt you are consuming naturally. Secondly, the salt you are adding to food, and thirdly, the large amounts of salt added to processed foods. The famous Australian, Vegemite, promoted for its B Vitamins, has an extremely high salt content.

According to The Australian Food Report, the average Australian breakfast cereal or loaf of bread is well above guidelines in sodium content. A third of all salt intake in the average Australian diet comes from breads and other cereals. *17*

For healthy cells, sodium, or salt, must be kept in balance with potassium. Sodium and potassium work together to maintain the right pressure of cellular fluids, inside and outside the cells. Too much sodium stops the potassium from doing its job. For a correct balance between sodium and potassium, your intake of potassium should be five times more than that of sodium. Refined foods are high in sodium and low in potassium. Examples of these foods are the refined processed foods, like table salt, processed cheese, beef cubes, bacon, soy sauce and Cornflakes. An excess of sodium has disruptive and even cancer-inducing effects inside the cell. It affects the water balance of the body and causes stress, fatigue and even depression. We therefore need to major on foods high in potassium but low in sodium. Examples of these foods are lentils, dried beans and peas, potatoes, nuts, bananas, green leafy vegetables, brown rice, carrots and apples. *18*

Max Gerson, an expert in dietary treatment of cancer in the 1900's, believed that the beginnings of all chronic illness lie in the sodium-potassium imbalance in body chemistry. Not only is potassium an important nerve conductor, but it acts as a catalyst for many body enzymes and is essential for proper muscle contraction, including muscles of the heart and those involved in digestion. Potassium also encourages good cell respiration and oxygenation. A sufficient oxygen supply to the cells is another important factor in the prevention of cancer. *19*

Cakes

Is it possible to make a healthy cake? Cakes that are made from unrefined flour, cold-pressed olive oil or coconut oil instead of margarine, and honey or fruit juice concentrate instead of sugar, are an improvement on the average homemade cake. However, there is still one remaining problem. Most cakes require baking powder, a component of self-raising flour, for a light consistency. Baking powder is not good for us, as it can contain heavy metals like aluminium. Baking powder also interferes with digestion in the stomach and inhibits the absorption of iron. If you are going to use baking powder occasionally, then choose a baking powder from a health shop. This will at least be free from heavy metals. Eggs or egg whites can be used as rising agents instead of baking powder, but these cakes will be fairly heavy in consistency. Slices and cookies on the other hand can be made successfully without baking powder. Cake recipes in this book are healthier than most cakes, but still not recommended as part of the 'diet for cancer patients' in *Chapter 7*.

Bread

It is important to look for 'good' bread. What is good bread? It is one made from wholesome flour and does not contain harmful additives. The emulsifiers, 471 and

472 are animal fats, often pig fat, and should be avoided. The food additive 282 should also be avoided. This is a mould inhibitor that gives stale goods a fresh look. It is reported to cause hyperactivity, aggression and learning difficulties in children. Allergic reactions include disturbance to upper gastrointestinal tract, migraine and headaches. [20]

Read all the labels carefully when buying and you will find some that don't contain these food additives. Organic sour rye-dough bread is one. 'Good bread' should also be low in salt and free from preservatives.

Live yeast is used in the making of all bread, so you should allow 24 hours after baking before eating. This gives sufficient time for the yeast to become inactive. Live yeast promotes the growth of candida, which is naturally occurring in the body but causes problems when it over-populates the gut.

Health shops can advise you on the best brands to buy. Organic sour-rye dough bread is a good option, but if you are battling with disease, brown rice is a better form of carbohydrate than bread.

Spices

Hot, spicy foods aggravate the lining of the stomach and can cause stomach ulcers and stomach cancer. A good alternative to pepper and chili powder is Hungarian Sweet Paprika, which is made from capsicum not chili.

Artificial colourings and flavourings

These have a variety of harmful effects such as hyperactivity in children, allergies and cancer. You can buy a decoder, or pamphlet, listing food additive numbers and their effects, as well as the general safety level of additives. However if you eat a diet of purely natural, unprocessed food you won't need a decoder.

Just to shock you into bypassing those 'special treats', here are the details on three common food colourings:

The following carcinogens are contained in a leading brand of chocolate sandwich biscuits, made in Australia for Australians, because the ingredients are banned in the USA and the E.U.

102 – Acid yellow or coal tar. 80% of hyperactive children are allergic to it. It is believed to cause allergic reactions in 15% of the general population. Known effects are asthma, hyperactivity, hay fever, blurred vision, breathing problems, skin irritation, wakefulness in young children.
110 – sunset yellow – toxic waste from petro-chemical industry and a known carcinogen.

129 – Allura Red colouring - a coal tar dye. It may cause allergic skin conditions. It increases the heart's rate and is implicated in behavioral problems. Persons suffering from asthma should avoid it. Listed problems associated with Allura Red are tumours and lymphoma. When given to mice, they developed cancer of the lymph glands.

A long-standing popular cherry-flavoured chocolate confectionery contains not only 102, 110 and 129 but also the red food colouring 123. And what's wrong with 123?

123 - Amaramth (Red food colouring) – All women of childbearing age, especially those in the first 3 months of pregnancy should avoid this colour. It may provoke eczema, is harmful to asthmatics and causes hyperactivity. It has caused birth defects and foetal deaths in some test animals. Implanted in mice bladders it produced cancer. As of October 1999 the ANZFA has allowed this chemical to be used either in large amounts and/or in more foods.[21]

Potentially dangerous colourings: 102; 104; 107; 110; 122-128; 133 and 155

And what's really in those artificial flavours?
- 'Cherry' – Aldehyde C17 – an aniline dye used in plastic and rubber.
- 'Vanilla' – Piperonal – a chemical used to kill lice.
- 'Pineapple' - Ethyl acetate – cleans leather, and its vapours are known to cause

chronic lung, liver and heart damage.
- 'Nut' – Butylaldehyde – used in rubber cement.
- 'Banana' – Amyl acetate – a paint solvent.
- 'Strawberry' – Benzyl acetate – a nitrate solvent.

Potentially dangerous flavourings: 621-623 and anything listed as 'flavouring'. (Artificial flavours don't have to be disclosed). [22]

Artificial sweeteners

Aspartame, also known as 'Nutrasweet', or food additive no. 951, contains Aspartic acid and Methanol. Aspartic acid can cause brain damage, and Methanol breaks down to formaldehyde, which spreads throughout the vital organs. Aspartame can trigger or mimic many diseases, including A.D.D., epilepsy, fibromyalgia, lupus and M.S. Aspartame is the sweetener in diet drinks, such as Diet Coke, and is the sweetener in most 'sugar-free' sweets and chewing gum. [23]

Preservatives

Some preservatives are labelled as 'antioxidants'. Most of us are aware of the wonderful health benefits of antioxidants. However there are good antioxidants and bad antioxidants. Antioxidants like grape seed and Vitamin E are free-radical scavengers, protecting us from cancer. However, certain preservatives in foods, labelled as antioxidants, can be detrimental to our health.

Examples of bad anti-oxidants are:
- BHA (butylated hydroxyanisole) – 320

This additive may cause dermatitis, asthma skin blisters, weakness, fatigue and cancer; a defoamer and stabiliser and is pesticide inert. Derived from Coal Tar Dye, it is reported to be the most widely used additive in the U.S. It is listed as a carcinogen and suspected of being a neurotoxin. It raises cholesterol levels in the blood and can cause hyperactivity.
- BHT (butylated hydroxytoluene) – 321 – similar effects to BHA. [24]

Sulphites – 220, 221 and 222 – these are a group of sulfur-based chemicals, also widely used as antioxidants in foods. As many as 1 in 100 people, according to the FDA are extremely sensitive to sulphites and may have difficulty in breathing, develop hives, diarrhoea, abdominal pain, cramps and dizziness, wheezing and vomiting. Sulphites are commonly used in cooked chips and preserved meats. [25]

Potentially dangerous preservatives: 210-213; 220-228; 250-252

According to ''The Australian and New Zealand Food Additive Decoder' all of the afore-mentioned additives have been classified as potentially dangerous, meaning that they may cause hyperactivity, anti-social behaviour, short attention span, lack of muscle co-ordination, skin disorders, asthma and allergies.

Chocolate

Cocoa contains caffeine, which can be addictive. Caffeine depletes the body of vitamins, especially B vitamins, essential for correct cell division. It also depletes potassium and magnesium levels in the body. Cocoa is produced in countries where there is often inadequate storage. The raw product lies in the open for months with rats and other rodents living in it. There are 'acceptable' levels of animal faeces and dead animals in cocoa. [26]

Cocoa and chocolate are prepared from the toxic residue left after the extraction of the highly valued cocoa butter. Tests on cattle, chickens and even the soil have shown cocoa residue to be poisonous. Chocolate has been associated with such allergic reactions as skin disorders, headaches, gastrointestinal symptoms, respiratory problems and nose bleeding. Cocoa contains theobromine, a nerve poison. An indulgence in chocolate may induce conditions that may be attributed to nerve disorders.[27]

However, some studies on chocolate, published in the American Journal of Clinical Nutrition March 2005, suggest that cocoa may actually be beneficial in regulating insulin levels and lowering blood pressure. This is due to the fact that cocoa can be rich in flavonols. (This will depend on the flavonol content of the plant it's derived from,)

However only properly processed chocolate can provide any health benefits, and the processing methods of chocolate today, destroy about one-quarter to one-half of chocolate's flavonols. Dark chocolate may have some antioxidant properties, whereas adding milk cancels out the chocolate's antioxidant effects, so milk chocolate and white chocolate definitely won't contain these beneficial nutrients. Dark chocolate still contains large quantities of sugar, and eating sugar is a profoundly negative influence on your immune system. If you are sick, you should be avoiding sugar altogether.

You do not have to eat chocolate to obtain the benefits of flavonols. Flavonols are found in fruits like apples, blueberries and grapes and almost all vegetables, including broccoli, greens and onions. These have other chemicals like anthocyanins that are even more powerful than the flavonols in cocoa in protecting against free-radical damage.[28]

Beverages

Pure water is best for cleansing the system. If you feel like the occasional warm drink, then a cup of pure herbal tea can be a substitute for traditional tea and coffee. Many herbal teas are beneficial, while traditional tea and coffee contain caffeine and tannin, both of which undermine the efficiency of the liver and kidneys. Caffeine is also consumed in the form of chocolate drinks and cola soft drinks. Other detrimental effects of caffeine include increased blood pressure and blood cholesterol levels, increased heart rate, stomach acidity and over-stimulation of the nervous system and adrenal glands. This may lead to anxiety, irritability, insomnia, heart palpitations, rapid breathing, heart disease, stomach ulcers, toxic effects upon a foetus, decreased iron absorption, increased loss of calcium and magnesium. Carbonated beverages should be avoided as they deplete the body's calcium stores, as they are required to neutralise the phosphoric acid component.

Most of us are aware of the importance of water. You die after just three days without it! However many people are under the misconception, that if they drink tea, coffee and soft drinks, they are getting enough water, because these drinks contain water. These drinks are actually diuretic in their effect. That means they are water-expelling, because their mostly acidic compositions require the body to give up water in order to eliminate their harmful residues. Dr. Batmanghelidj did some outstanding work on the therapeutic value of water. He says that for every cup of regular tea or coffee you drink, you need to make up for it by drinking a glass of water.

Dr. Batmanghelidj, as a political prisoner in a Tehran prison, cured other prisoners by using water alone. He treated prisoners with water alone, because that was all he had available. Later, after escaping to the U.S., he was able to continue his research. Dr. Batmanghelidj proved that water does have therapeutic value, and that dehydration creates the foundation for many diseases.

Water is essential for brain function, bone function, nerve function, and is intricately involved in the body's water-dependent chemical reactions. It is required for cellular energy, digestion, detoxification and for maintaining the right blood pH level. The body uses water to buffer acidity. Lack of it creates all manner of illnesses, including allergies, depression, heartburn and ulcers. Most of the population have become chronically and dangerously dehydrated due to the decision that water is too bland to drink, and needs replacing with tea, coffee and carbonated beverages.[29]

One should drink between meals but not with meals. Drinking with meals interferes with digestion by dilution of the digestive juices. It is also best to start the day with 2 glasses of water, or warm water with a slice of lemon. The body needs plenty of liquid for cleansing and flushing the system. Adults need to drink at least 6-8 glasses of water per day. Children and the elderly need to be reminded to drink as they often forget.

The acid-alkaline balance

We need 20-30% acid-forming foods, and 70-80% alkaline-forming foods per day, depending on how quickly a person burns up their calories.

Acid-forming foods: all flesh foods, all dairy foods, sugar, eggs, grains, baked foods, pasta, legumes, tomatoes, bananas, oranges, grapefruit, plums.

Alkaline-forming foods: all fruits and vegetables except for those previously mentioned, sprouts, fresh raw nuts, dates, seeds, fresh raw vegetable juices, noni juice, green barley/spirulina powder, green tea, olive oil. Raw plant foods are better for alkalising than cooked plant foods.[30]

Endnotes

1. Cilento, R., *Heal Cancer: Choose your own survival path*, Aust.,1993, p. 157
2. Heathman, L., & Tillotson, A., *Leaves From the Tree of Life*, U.S.A., 1996, p. 6.8
3. Martin, G., *Lifestyle Excellence, The Fat Family*, April-June 04
4. *Well Being Magazine* no. 65 p. 69
5. Martin, G., op. cit.
6. Ibid
7. Ford, D., *Worth More Than A Million*, U.S.A. 1987, p. 83
8. Hollingsworth, E., *Take Control of Your Health*, Aust., 2002, p. 292
9. Leggett, M. & S., *The Australian Food Report*, Aust., 1989, p. 76.
10. Taubert, P.M., *Your Health and Food Additives*, Aust., 2000, p. 47
11. Ford, op. cit., p. 83
12. Lee, Dr. J., *Hormonal Balance* audio C.D.
13. Leggett, op.cit., p. 8
14. Hollingsworth, E., op. cit., pp. 293-294
15. Heathman & Tillotson, op.cit., p. 2.7
16. De Langre, Jacques, (biochemist), *Sea Salt's Hidden Powers*
17. Legget. op. cit., p. 94
18. Woollams, C. *The Tree of Life*, U.K. 2004, pp. 23-25
19. Ibid
20. Taubert, P.M. *Your Health and Food Additives*, Aust 2000
21. Ibid
22. Reekie, Lillian, *Hidden Dangers*, 2002, Aust.
23. Taubert, P.M., op Cit.
24. Ibid
25. Ibid
26. Woollams, C., *The Tree of Life*, 2004, p. 40
27. Craig, W.J., *Nutrition for the Nineties*, U.S.A., pp. 288 & 360

28. Mercola, J., *The Total Health Program, Should You Eat Chocolate?* March 23, 2005
29. Day, P., *Water, The Stuff of Life*, Credence U.K., 2004, pp. 15-19
30. Woollams, op. cit., pp. 229-230

chapter three

the BEST foods to EAT

Plant foods are the best foods. A well-balanced, predominantly plant-based diet, will not only meet your nutritional needs, but at the same time will protect you from cancer, heart disease, salmonella and diseases passed on by animals. Plant foods, especially raw, can build your immune system and build your body's resistance to the increasing number of viral diseases of this century. You will come down with fewer colds, and if you do happen to catch the flu, your immune system will be able to fight it off before it develops into something serious.

Proteins

The recommended level of protein required by the human body is now known to be far less than considered necessary 50 years ago…and yet Western Society is eating far more meat. Too much protein places too much strain on the digestive system. A high protein diet leads to an acidic system, which causes calcium to be leached from the bones. This is the body's own defence mechanism for rebalancing the pH. A diet with a high proportion of meat and dairy products provides more protein than the body can cope with. *1*

Consider eating plant foods to acquire the recommended intake of protein. Some plant foods to eat for protein are whole grains, lentils, fruit, vegetables and nuts.

Having too little protein in the diet can also be a problem, particularly for growing children who may not eat a wide variety of plant foods. Adding some free-range eggs or mercury-free fish can provide some additional protein.

Starches

Starches should account for most of your daily calories, but avoid refined starches.

Plant foods for starch: whole grains, lentils, dried beans, sweet potatoes, bananas and many other fruits and vegetables.

Fats

Nuts, seeds, fruits and vegetables are excellent sources of fats and oils. Avocado is particularly good. So is coconut oil. Avocado can be used as a spread on sandwiches, included in salads, and goes well with potatoes. Coconut oil can be added to fruit smoothies, added to muesli, and to hot rice for a Thai flavour. It can be used in home-made sweet treats like truffles and slices.

Mercury-free fish and fish-oils are excellent for vitamin D and essential fatty acids. These are important for brain function and help prevent cancer and heart disease. Fish oils are high in the omega-3 fatty acid, which helps keep the balance with omega-6 fatty acids, essentially found in plant foods. Plant foods high in beneficial oils: nuts, seeds, many fruits and vegetables, particularly avocado and coconuts.

Sugars

We get all the sugar we need from fruit and vegetables. If you need to sweeten any food you are making yourself, use fruit juice concentrate or natural cold-extracted honey. Refined table sugar, brown or white should be avoided due to the stress it places upon the immune system. When calculating your daily sugar intake, remember to take into account sugar added to processed foods!

Vitamins and minerals

For maximum nutrition, fruit and vegetables should be fresh, organic and raw, or as close to raw as possible.

Plant foods for vitamins and minerals: fruits, vegetables, whole grains and legumes.

Plant foods for calcium, listed in order of calcium content: brazil nuts, spinach, chick peas, broccoli, sesame seeds, lentils, figs, blackberries, apricots, green beans, cherries, parsley, cabbage, pumpkin.

Plant foods for iron: bran, wholegrains, spirulina, pepitas or pumpkin seeds, wheat germ, sunflower seeds, parsley, potato, raw cabbage, beetroot, peas and many other vegetables.

Remember to include vitamin B12 in the diet for iron absorption. This can be in supplement form, or from free-range eggs, organic yoghurt, organic meat, mercury-free fish or fish-oil. For those undertaking the 'diet for cancer patients', Max Gerson recommends no animal protein at all in the first four months, but to take a vitamin B12 supplement instead. *(See Chapter 7.)*

Foods that help with the absorption of iron are those containing vitamin C, vitamin E, calcium and folic acid. Vitamin C is found in many fruits and vegetables including citrus, berries, apples, cabbage, cauliflower, spinach and parsley. Vitamin E is found in cold-pressed olive oil, sunflower seeds, nuts, wholegrains, dark green vegetables and eggs. Folic acid is found in green leafy vegetables. Consuming foods made with baking powder decreases your body's ability to absorb the iron. [2]

Endnotes

1. Ford, D., *Worth More Than A Million*, U.S.A., 1987, p. 83
2. Xandria Williams, *Iron Essentials, Well Being Magazine* No. 61 pp. 52-54

chapter four

PRACTICAL aspects of EATING for HEALTH

Getting the family off junk food

The first step is to convince your family that they need to replace unhealthy food with healthy alternatives. If they understand the reasons for doing so, and if they are convinced of the facts, then they will be more willing to change. Each family member should try to have a good mental attitude and a sense of adventure. Discovering new foods will involve change. Things may taste a little different for a while, but by supporting each other in this change, junk food will soon be a thing of the past. Persevere! It's worth it!

Be consistent. If you have decided to come off junk food, don't indulge even occasionally. Never allow junk food to enter your supermarket trolley. This doesn't mean that your family will miss out on treats. It just means that you, as the family cook, will have to work hard at finding substitute treats.

There are many recipes in this book that will fill the junk food gap. You just need to experiment to find out what appeals to your family. Keep the larder stocked with fruit and healthy homemade snacks. If there's nothing else to eat, then the family will gradually learn to accept what is available.

Milk substitutes

Eliminating dairy milk may be difficult. Rice, nut and oat milks are good alternatives. These can be homemade in a blender. If buying rice milk or oat milk, look for a brand with no added cane sugar and without canola oil. Organic non-homogenised goat's milk can be bought from some health shops. This is more digestible than cow's milk, and may be an option for young children. Organic natural yoghurt is another option for children.

Use the blender to make 'milk' shakes. Add favourite fruits to rice milk and blend. Vitamin and mineral supplements may be blended into to the 'milk' shake.

Living with less meat

Cutting down the amount of meat in your diet may seem like a challenge. I started by choosing some favourite dishes in which animal foods could be substituted with plant foods. I chose spaghetti bolognaise and lamb stew. Instead of using all minced steak in the bolognaise, I used 50% brown lentils and 50% minced steak. The rest of the ingredients remained the same. I did the same with the lamb stew. I used 50% lamb and 50% kidney beans (or sometimes white beans). As these two recipes gained success I gradually increased the plant-food content and removed the meat. Another recipe I tried was meat pie. Instead of using all minced steak, I used 50% brown lentils. Our meat pie gradually became lentil pie. Legumes, (lentils, dried peas and beans), are a wonderful staple food. Once you have learned to cook them you will find them easier to cook than meat, very tasty and so economical! Many people think that the only way to eat lentils is in the form of lentil soup. However this is not the only way to eat them. You can prepare lentils as a thick lentil stew, served on a plate with salad and vegetables - not just a few lentils floating around the bottom of a bowl of soup.

Butter or margarine?

This is the question that has been debated for years. Both can present problems. Margarine affects liver function, damages arteries and is highly carcinogenic. Butter contains pesticides, hormones and a whole host of toxins, because toxins are stored in the fat cells of the animal.

When we decided to 'go healthy', butter and margarine were the first items we deleted from our diet, and quite honestly, we didn't miss them. This was because of the wonderful recipe, Savoury Cashew Spread *(see recipe section)*, which really is an excellent substitute for butter and cheese.

It is amazing how many people automatically spread every slice of bread with butter or margarine, regardless of the filling or topping. Salad sandwiches do not need butter/margarine if you use avocado. Commercial nut spreads, like hazelnut spread, as well as tahini, are also good options. Most children actually don't mind having spreads placed directly on the bread or toast. For cooking purposes, ground nuts, cold-pressed olive oil or coconut oil can replace butter in slices and pastries. A little organic butter occasionally can also be used.

What's your label?

Many people are hung up about being vegetarian or vegan. The important thing is to eat for health, and not be bound to the restraints of a label. A vegetarian does not eat meat, but their diet may not be healthy, because they simply replace meat with cheese, and don't even eliminate food additives. A vegan, by definition, can still eat food additives. Vegans who don't supplement may have health problems caused by low iron and lack of vitamin B12. We believe that the healthiest way to go is to choose foods that are as organic and as close to nature as possible, with a predominance of plant foods, and a small amount of clean animal products. However, if you are undertaking the 'diet for cancer patients', *(Chapter 7)*, then it is vital to go without any animal products for 4 months.

Suggestions for school lunches and picnics

Apart from sandwiches, which may become boring, there are many interesting possibilities. Many children like snack foods. For school lunches, you can prepare your own health snacks, like raw carrot, sultanas and pumpkin seeds all in small packages. Rice cakes are also a favourite. They can be spread with nut spread, or just eaten plain. Any of the snacks, slices or cakes from the recipe section are excellent for lunches. For example, pizza, made from pita bread and topped with Savoury Cashew Spread instead of cheese, is popular with children. It doesn't have to be served hot.

Some children prefer hot food, especially in winter, and can be accommodated with a flask of soup or lentils. Hot savoury rice and vegetables, steamed vegetables and split pea soup all go well in a flask.

Suggestions for children's birthday parties

Most children come to a birthday party expecting to eat junk food. However I was pleasantly surprised at the popularity of the more healthy food I served at my own children's birthday parties.

Fruit sorbet, made in a centrifuge juicer or Thermomix is great. A decorative platter of fresh fruit looks very attractive, as do canned fruits in glass bowls. Because children usually have preferences for certain fruits, different canned fruits in separate bowls may be better than mixing them together as a fruit salad. The muffins made from recipes in this book are usually popular as are pancakes or waffles made in a waffle maker. Low-salt corn chips, available from health shops, are not too bad for special occasions and not too expensive. You can also make your own popcorn. Fruit juice is a better option than soft drink and not much more expensive.

The social question

Before allowing ourselves to be considered anti-social, we must remember that the nutritional understanding of our whole society is severely lacking. The whole culinary culture of Western society is based on wrong principles. Let's face it! All that hydrogenated oil, white flour, cream, cheese, sugar and meat are hardly doing us any good! In fact, many poorer cultures produce a far healthier population. The traditional Asian diet, consisting of mainly rice and vegetables, only a little meat and no dairy products, is far healthier than the Western diet. Statistics on cancer and heart disease in our own culture during the Great Depression show lower incidence of these diseases. This was because people were forced to do without products like butter, cream and even meat during these years. Realising the inherent problems of the Western diet, we have to find the balance between eating a healthy diet and remaining socially acceptable.

What about the Aussie barbeque?

Being invited to a barbeque can be a bit difficult if you don't eat meat. I usually steam some potatoes whole, in their jackets. I then wrap them in a layer of baking paper followed by a layer of foil. This prevents the aluminium from coming into contact with the potato. We can then just throw the potatoes on the barbeque. They only need to heat through so they don't take very long. The same can be done with sweet corn. Who can go past a meal of potatoes-in-jackets and sweet corn served with delicious salads!

What about eating out?

We do not often eat out at restaurants, but for special occasions, we try to make healthy choices from the menu. All restaurants serve salad and steamed vegetables. These should be looked upon as the basis of the meal rather than the 'additional extra'. One can always ask for larger servings of these in place of the meat dish. When invited to the homes of friends I usually bring something along to share. It is important to reassure your host that 'health fanatics' really only eat ordinary food, like salads, vegetables, rice and fruits.

When attending a function where it is a 'bring and share' arrangement, I usually prepare a very large casserole and a salad as well. This provides a healthy choice for both my own family and others. Examples of popular casserole dishes are Layered Vegetable Casserole, Red Lentil Lasagne and Spiced Chick Peas. It's amazing how many people will ask you for the recipe.

What about guests?

Catering for guests who are not accustomed to healthy food is no real problem. Even though many think that healthy food consists of strange concoctions, it is important to remember that rice, vegetables and salad are very acceptable to the average person. Guests will enjoy any of the soups, pasta and vegetable casseroles, vegetable lasagne, and probably any of the 'treats for special occasions' in Part B of this book. For guests who enjoy dairy milk in traditional tea, you can keep small servings of milk in the freezer, in small plastic containers or ice-cube trays. Individual portions of frozen milk can be thawed very quickly, by standing the container in hot water. For afternoon tea, waffles and pancakes, served with pure maple syrup, fruit or fruit sorbet are a great success.

Isn't healthy food expensive?

When someone says, "I could never afford to be on a healthy diet", they really mean:
"I could never afford to buy healthy foods in addition to the food I am currently eating."

Let's get one thing straight! The healthiest foods available, namely fruit, vegetables, lentils, pulses and brown rice, are not expensive! Other healthy foods may be comparatively expensive, but they are not always necessary. The thing we must remember is that when changing to a healthy diet we are actually minimising some of the most expensive foods. Meat is one of the most expensive food items. So are cheese, butter and commercial ice creams. Also consider the cost of packaged breakfast cereals, commercially produced biscuits, cakes and muesli bars. As for junk foods, they are a complete waste of money, whatever the cost, because they are nutritionally deficient! If we avoid these foods, then we can afford to buy the more expensive health foods like nuts, avocados and cold-pressed olive oil.

If you were on a very low budget, you couldn't do better than majoring on fruits, vegetables, seeds, legumes and brown rice. In changing to such a diet you would actually be getting much better value for money. On a global scale, if we all ate plant foods, there would be much more food to go around. For example, 40,000 pounds of potatoes can be harvested from one acre in comparison to 250 pounds of beef. *1*

Isn't healthy cooking, time consuming?

There is no doubt that preparing your own food will take longer than opening packets and cans. The convenience foods available to us today make it all too tempting to save time on food preparation. When people say, "I haven't the time", they usually mean, "It's not a priority". We always make time for things that are a priority.

Changing to a healthy cooking style takes some adjustment, but once you have taken the step and learned a new routine, it's no more difficult or time consuming than the way you used to cook. Careful planning, foresight and the use of modern kitchen appliances can cut down on preparation time immensely.

Let's compare these two spaghetti sauces: one is vegetarian and one is meat based. We'll look at the time and effort involved in preparing each.

Spaghetti Sauce (meat version)
1. Remember to take the meat out of the freezer the night before.
2. Blend tomatoes, tomato paste and onions in blender.
3. Stir-fry the minced steak in fry pan until brown. Drain off excess fat.
4. Add the meat to the prepared tomato sauce and cook in a large pot for about 2 hours.
5. Scrub the fatty pot vigorously with a scourer. Likewise, scrub fry-pan.

Spaghetti Sauce (lentil version)
1. Remember to soak lentils overnight, rinse them and put them in the crock-pot with water next morning.
2. Blend tomatoes, tomato paste and onions in blender.
3. Half an hour before the meal, transfer cooked lentils to a large pot, with the prepared tomato sauce.
4. Cook for half and hour.
5. Give the cooking pot and crock-pot a quick wash.

The vegetarian meal eliminates the need to pre-fry meat and reduces the clean up time, due to the lower fat content of the dish. The use of a crock-pot vastly cuts down on the effort involved in cooking lentils. Both meals involve a certain amount of thinking ahead. For the lentil version you have to remember to soak the lentils, while the meat version involves remembering to thaw the meat. Which do you think required the most time and effort to prepare?

Now you might be thinking that the steak in the fry pan and the steamed vegetables still takes the prize for the least preparation, but such a diet can become boring, and meat day after day is not the healthiest way to go.

Just because a dish is vegetarian does not necessarily mean that it will take more time to prepare. The time factor in preparing food depends on the type of dish, whether vegetarian or non-vegetarian. Some meat dishes take a lot of preparation. Think about the roast with baked potatoes...all that slaving over a hot oven...the turning of the food, and the big mess at the end!

Eating away from home

At some stage, most of us will be in a situation where we cannot cook for our family because we are away from our kitchen conveniences. This situation may arise while on holidays. In this situation, what is the best 'ready-to-eat' food we can buy? Eating at a good restaurant may be an option, but will be expensive. Fast foods on the other hand may be cheaper, but will not be at all healthy. The supermarket is a good alternative to the fast food store. Many supermarkets are open 24 hours a day, 7 days a week.

I have found the following 'ready-to-eat' foods to be the best alternatives to fast foods. When going on holidays, it pays to pack plastic plates, cutlery and a can opener for eating 'on the road'.
- All fruits
- Salad vegetables, including avocado if ripe
- 'Good' bread or pita bread
- Rice cakes
- Muesli with rice milk or grape juice
- Dried fruits and nuts

- Nut spread
- Canned beans
- Eggs
- Canned wild salmon

A small gas stove is a good investment for 'eating on the road', and a small electric saucepan is useful for heating canned food in situations where you have access to power but no stove.

Canned foods without additives are useful in such situations. Many people think that all foods with a long shelf-life contain preservatives. However, preserving by means of bottling and canning are techniques that have been practiced for years. The food lasts because of the absence of air rather than the addition of preservatives. Of course some canned foods do contain preservatives and additives, but many do not. Read the labels carefully.

Will a predominantly plant-based diet give me enough strength?

Anyone who is serious about nutrition needs to consider a predominantly whole-food, plant-food diet, minimising meat and dairy products.

Consider the staying power of the ox, the horse, the camel and the elephant. These are all vegetarian animals. On the other hand, lions and tigers have short periods of intense energy but do not have endurance. Consumption of substantial amounts of meat reduces our energy reserves due to the great tax it places on the digestive system. [2]

Edwin Moses, an Olympic gold medallist who competed in the 400-metre hurdles for eight years without losing a single race, was a vegetarian. Dave Scott, also a vegetarian, won the Hawaii Ironman Triathlon four times. Daniel from the Bible, who refused the rich food from the king's table and ate only vegetables, was in very good health.

Will a predominantly plant-based diet give me enough protein?

As the years have passed, scientists have been making lower and lower estimates of the daily need for protein. Nuts, seeds and legumes are all good sources of protein. For those who are taking on the 'diet for cancer patients', and excluding animal products, it is important to include at least one source of plant protein at every meal. It is also important to eat a wide variety of foods. After the initial few months of excluding animal products, it can be helpful to add a small amount of clean organic animal products, due to the risk of vitamin B12 and iron deficiency. For vegetarians who include eggs, there is no risk of lacking vitamin B12. [3]

Should thin people eat a predominantly plant-based diet?

Some people are genetically programmed to be thin. They have a high metabolic rate, which means that they use energy quickly. It is important for thin people especially, to include plenty of the good fats. This is particularly important with children. Avocados, olive oil, coconut oil, nut spreads, tahini, ground linseeds, sesame seeds and sunflower seeds all provide good oils. Mercury-free fish oils and free-range eggs can be added to this list.

Thin people are more prone to osteoporosis, so particular care needs to be taken to ensure adequate calcium/magnesium intake from plant foods. A calcium/magnesium supplement may also be advisable.

Can supplements compensate for a diet of junk food?

Vitamins, minerals and medicinal herbs are most effective when combined with a healthy eating pattern. Vitamin supplements can provide additional nutrients, but the benefits will be compromised by the consumption of foods that overload the immune system. Sugar for example, depletes the body's stores of vitamins and minerals. All vitamins should be taken in a balanced formula – not separately – and should be taken in conjunction with a colloidal mineral supplement. Minerals are catalysts for chemical reactions in the body, and vitamins will only work for you if minerals are present. Vitamins and minerals must be from an organic plant source, and scientifically proven to absorb into the cells. Many cheaper brands pass straight through the system, with very little absorption.

Is it possible for me to change?

There are many who say, "I've eaten this way all my life. It's too late to change now." While it is true that children under twelve years of age adapt more easily to a change in diet, it is not impossible for others to change. Be convinced about the need for change. Make small gradual changes. Start with just one change, adding one more change each new week. Try to be consistent, but don't be discouraged by your failures.

Endnotes

1. Virkler, M. & P., *Go Natural*, U.S.A. 1995, p. 45
2. Ford, D., *Worth More Than A Million*, U.S.A., 1987, p.83.
3. *The Lancet* medical journal, November 1959

chapter five

COPING with CANCER

My husband had been suffering from chronic fatigue for a number of years. He also suffered from colds and chest infections, which lingered on for months, sometimes requiring up to five courses of antibiotics to regain health.

In December 1996 Paul went for a CT scan that showed probable lymphoma, a cancer of the lymphatic system. Although suffering from a persistent cough, and in no condition to undergo surgery, Paul was strongly urged by the specialist to undergo diagnostic surgery as soon as possible. This was to find out the exact type of lymphoma so that appropriate treatment could be given.

We were given much confidence by the specialist, who assured us that 90% of all lymphoma cases are completely curable through chemotherapy. Because most cases of lymphoma are aggressive, and fast moving, diagnostic surgery seemed fairly urgent. This would involve removal of some lymph nodes deep down within the abdomen, which we were told would be a fairly 'tricky' operation.

Shortly after Christmas we were given the name of a health retreat in Queensland, run by naturopaths. The retreat, Living Valley Springs, offered short-term live-in sessions involving fasting, colonic cleansing and natural therapy. At the same time we were reading as much information as we could get our hands on about natural therapy.

Despite strong opposition from the cancer specialist, Paul decided to cancel his diagnostic operation, scheduled for January, and instead go for nine days of natural therapy. On returning home, there was no sign of the cough, and Paul felt much rejuvenated. As he continued with a strict diet and food supplements, as recommended by Living Valley Springs, his health continued to improve. We were gaining more and more confidence in natural therapy. We were also greatly encouraged by our local naturopath who supplied herbal tonics and much valuable information.

Additionally, Paul received prayer, a powerful experience that gave him faith. This was to be a great source of encouragement later, when he experienced times of despair and depression. Each time of depression presented a battle, which Paul had to fight with determination, holding on to the promise of life through faith in God, rather than focusing on the prospect of terminal illness.

Later in February Paul had a call, out of the blue, from the oncologist who explained that it was imperative that Paul submit himself for diagnostic surgery because there was a strong chance that the lymphoma was aggressive. Paul finally decided to go for the surgery. He was now feeling much stronger and able to face it. The surgery involved seven days in hospital, five of those days on an intravenous drip of saline solution. This was a fairly traumatic experience but Paul made a good recovery. He returned immediately to the strict diet and supplements.

Two weeks after the surgery we were called to discuss the results. Much to everyone's surprise, Paul was not in the 90% of 'curable' lymphoma cases. He had a rarer type of non-Hodgkin's lymphoma, (small-cell follicular), for which there was, at that time, no medical 'cure'. Chemotherapy and radiotherapy were ineffective on this type of cancer. The cancer was said to be fairly slow growing, which meant Paul had approximately four to seven years to live.

Instead of being shocked by the news, we were relieved. By this time we had done enough research on natural therapy to know that chemotherapy and radiotherapy were not the only way. In fact we were relieved to be free from making the decision on which way to go. Because Paul's cancer was slow growing, it meant that there was time for natural therapy to work. We also believed in the healing power of a mighty God who was working for us!

We continued to believe that God would heal by both natural and supernatural means. Natural therapy meant obedience to a strict healthy diet and taking of the best nutritional supplements we could find. Making use of all the healing properties in God's creation played as much importance as our overall belief that God would heal.

The first year proved to be the most difficult. Keeping hope and faith alive was not always easy, but vital. We discovered that the way we spoke about the illness was important. It was often necessary to explain to people why we were eating the way we were, or why Paul didn't have enough energy to do things on certain days. Instead of saying, "I've got lymphoma", Paul trained himself to say, "I'm recovering from cancer."

Changing the diet for the whole family gave Paul encouragement and support. The children, at the ages of eight and ten years, were extremely cooperative. It was also extremely timesaving for me as the cook, because it meant that I didn't have to cook separate meals for Paul, who needed a non-meat diet for recovery. We all sat down to lentils, vegetables and salad together. (I did supplement the children's diet with some eggs and organic natural yoghurt.) Over the past eight years we have given advice and support to many cancer patients. The ones who have the best chance are those who have a supportive partner who can prepare food and juice in the appropriate way.

One year after diagnosis, Paul was no longer suffering from chronic fatigue. The occasional cold was thrown off within a week without resorting to antibiotics. Eighteen months after the diagnosis of the lymphoma, Paul decided to visit his cancer specialist to report his amazing good health. A physical examination showed that the spleen was quite normal and not swollen as it was previously. Neither was there any swelling of the lymph nodes. The specialist advised that there was no need for another CT scan, which involved some degree of exposure to radioactivity. The physical evidence was enough!

Four years after diagnosis we read about the value of taking apricot kernels for healing and prevention of cancer. In Phillip Day's book, Cancer, Why We're Still Dying to Know the Truth, we found testimonials of people who had been healed from cancer using natural therapy, part of that therapy being vitamin B17 found in apricot kernels. Paul started taking the kernels along with the important enzymes. Fresh pineapple provides the enzyme, bromelain, and fresh paw paw or papaya contains papain. These fruits are eaten for breakfast. Additional pancreatic enzymes are taken in tablet form. Paul took 30 kernels a day for six months, just to make sure that the cancer was really gone, and then continued on a maintenance dose of 14 per day. Many people think that apricot kernels are toxic, but this is not the case. The compound of cyanide they contain is different to actual cyanide, and is only toxic to cancer cells. *(See Chapter 8.)*

Eight years after diagnosis Paul is in good health and still continues to take a maintenance dose of 14 kernels per day. The diet and list of food supplements, given in chapter 7, may be of help to cancer patients. This is not meant to be a recipe for the healing of all cancer patients. No treatment works for everyone. It is important that each person intending to embark on natural therapy consults a good naturopath, and preferably attends a live-in cleanse centre such as Living Valley Springs. Most therapies treat the symptoms, and ignore the cause of the disease. If the cause is toxicity, then it must be eliminated, or the disease will return.

Finding the right path for treatment can be a difficult decision, but no one can go wrong with building the immune system and cutting down toxins, whatever therapy you choose. You will be bombarded with opinions from friends and family, but ultimately the decision is yours. Choose a treatment that makes the most sense to you, and if you choose natural therapy, go for it with all your might. Don't procrastinate. Be 100% committed and do everything you can to save your life. The ones who make it are the ones who are prepared to do everything possible. It will be costly in terms of time and money, but after all, it's your life, and what value can you put on a life?

chapter six

do WE really KNOW the CAUSE of CANCER?

Statistics now show that one in every three people in the U.S.A. will contract some kind of cancer at some time during their life. All western, affluent countries including Australia have similar statistics.[1]

To avoid cancer we need to maintain a healthy immune system. The immune system can be weakened by a combination of many factors: poor nutrition, toxic chemicals, emotional stress, allergies, moulds, pollens and yeast for example. A weakened immune system increases susceptibility to fatigue, bacteria and viral infection, depressions, headaches, allergies and cancer.

Diet

We can no longer doubt the direct link between diet and cancer. Although previously denied by orthodox medicine, the possibility became clear in 1982 when the US National Cancer Institute published a report summarising the evidence. As a result, scientists and doctors all around the world started to study the diet-cancer link. [2]

Some people who live on a diet of high protein, fat, sugar, salt, preservatives and artificial food additives can get away with it. Others, however will eventually become a victim of their poor eating habits. Because it is impossible to know whether or not we will be the susceptible one, it is safer for all to use common sense in eating habits.

Research shows that there is a direct link between high fat intake and cancer. People in affluent countries typically consume large amounts of rich foods like meat and dairy products, which are high in fat and low in fibre. Fat contributes to approximately 40% of calorie intake in these countries. People in poorer countries typically consume starchy foods as the basis to their diet. These foods are lower in fat and higher in fibre. Fat intake in these countries represents 10 - 20% of total calorie intake.

A trial involving 400 people from three capital cities in Australia showed that those who lowered their fat intake and increased fibre intake virtually eliminated the growth of large polyps in the bowel. All had been treated for bowel polyps previously. *3*

High fat and high protein go together. It seems that the affluent countries who consume such diets have a higher incidence of cancer. Statistics representing colon cancer deaths in 1975 showed Canada, New Zealand, USA, Australia, France and Switzerland as being the top six countries. El Salvador, Thailand, Colombia, Panama, Chile and Puerto Rico were the lowest. *4*

In 1983, a scientific study began on the dietary patterns in China. The study was done in 65 different counties, looking at the causes of death. The project found that certain groups of diseases tended to occur in similar economic and geographic areas. Diseases in "rich" areas included cancer, heart disease and osteoporosis, and correlated directly with high blood cholesterol and high nitrogen content in the urine. Diseases in "poor" areas included pneumonia and TB, but very little heart disease, cancer or osteoporosis. The conclusion drawn was that the diseases of affluence, found near the large Chinese cities, were directly linked to diets richer in animal products. These people had higher blood cholesterol, and higher urea nitrogen levels. Urea nitrogen is what is left over from the metabolism of protein in the body. The more of this we find in the blood, the higher our level of excess dietary protein. And, as the China Project data showed, the more animal products consumed, the more we are likely to take in more protein than we need. [5]

This may seem to conflict with the findings of Weston Price, who researched the traditional diets in the early 1900's. He found that people groups who ate traditional diets, whether vegetarian or animal based, did not contract cancer. However, the missing factor here was toxicity. As part of the China Project, a diet high in animal protein was fed to animals that had been exposed to cancer-causing toxins. Their livers developed tumours that grew rapidly. However, the tumours stopped growing when animal protein was decreased and replaced with plant protein. It appears that once the body has all the protein it needs, then the excess protein begins to feed pre-cancerous lesions and tumours.[6]

So, it seems that combining a diet high in animal products with a toxic environment is a recipe for cancer. Animal fat becomes contaminated with toxic residues as animals are exposed to environmental toxins. This is because toxins are stored in the fat cells. If we were in a completely pristine environment, with no stress, toxins or radiation, with soils that nourished the food it sustained, with a way of life geared to exercise, then it may be possible to eat a predominantly meat-based diet and still maintain good health. However, this is not possible today. We cannot transport the Weston Price research into the 21st century, because toxicity is affecting the whole planet. People who lived one hundred years ago also ate more raw foods – raw milk, raw fish, raw eggs. The enzymes in raw foods help protect against cancer, as do the enzymes in raw plant foods. Today it is not possible to consume raw animal foods because of the increase in bacterial diseases.

Modern-day farming practices, such as the use of artificial fertilizers, can be another cause of cancer. Fruit and vegetables now lack vitamins, minerals and antioxidants, and so will not give us the protection we need. Fortunately good supplements are available for those who decide to make up for the lack.

Environmental toxins

We live in an increasingly polluted world. Our food, homes, air and the water are becoming more and more toxic. As we are exposed to toxins, the body's defence mechanisms go into action. However, toxins may still build up to a point at which the body's cells can no longer cope.

The best way to avoid toxins in food is to eat unprocessed food. Many of the additives found in processed food do not have to be listed on packets. It's far less complicated to make your own food. It may take a little more time, but at least you know what you're eating.

If you were told that there were toxic chemicals in your home, what would come to mind... cleaning products? Insect sprays?

Most of us are aware of the toxicity of these, but few would suspect the bathroom to contain a whole host of toxic chemicals. Would you expect your shampoo, conditioner, deodorant, toothpaste and make-up to contain toxic cancer-causing ingredients? Most people wouldn't, trusting government protection agencies to ban anything that was toxic. But this is not the case.

Dr. Samuel Epstein, professor of environmental medicine and founder of the U.S. Cancer Prevention Coalition, says that health warnings similar to those found on cigarette packets should be placed on 'cancer-causing' cosmetics and toiletries. He says that there is overwhelming evidence on the presence of a wide range of carcinogens in cosmetics and personal care products.[7]

It is now known that the skin is a carrier, not a barrier. This means that substances get absorbed through the skin and carried to our organs. Many substances accumulate gradually in our liver and kidneys.

Most shampoos, bubble bath, shower gels and toothpaste contain a foaming agent called Sodium Lauryl Sulphate. This substance has over 90 different names, so unless a foaming product is labelled SLS free, then the foaming agent will be SLS, simply because it's cheap. SLS can form nitrates when it interacts with other substances. It goes in through the skin easily, allowing the penetration of other carcinogens. It can damage skin and can damage the immune system. *8*

Almost ALL hair conditioners, skin lotions and make-up contain a sliding agent called Propylene Glycol. This is another substance that is highly absorbable, and can also cause kidney and liver abnormalities.

Other toxins to watch out for in bathroom products are the chemicals, DEA, TEA, or anything with a capital E, formaldehyde, aluminium, toluene or fluoride. Hair sprays, nail polish, perfumes, deodorant, talc, make-up, and sunscreens all carry hidden dangers. Try to find a company that is committed to producing safe bathroom products, and be aware that the labelling of a product as natural, organic, or herbal may not necessarily be an indication of safety. A good website for understanding toxic chemicals is Samuel Epstein's site: www.preventcancer.com.au

Hormonal imbalance

Chemicals that we now encounter in every day life cause hormonal imbalance. These chemicals cause oestrogen dominance. This means low progesterone levels in women and low testosterone levels in men. Progesterone is a protective hormone. We need the right balance of progesterone or testosterone for protection against lifestyle diseases, and for a strong immune system. Our bodies absorb oestrogen mimics from pesticides, plastics, drugs, chemicals in personal care products, glues and household cleaning agents. The body recognises these as oestrogen.

The chemicals found in cheap plastics, are possibly the worst offenders. Much of our food, drink, toothpaste and shampoo are sold in these cheap plastic containers. We absorb these chemicals as they leach out of the bottle into the contents. We absorb oestrogen even by handling plastic wrap. Synthetic oestrogens, or oestrogen mimics, all cause oestrogen overload in our bodies. Animal fat consumption also increases oestrogen levels because the fat of the animal is the storage site for chemicals and hormones. *Hormone Replacement Therapy* and the *Pill* are a deadly source of oestrogen.

Many researchers are convinced that oestrogen dominance is responsible for the spreading of cancer in the body. Excess oestrogen, especially oestrogen mimics, have been clearly shown to weaken the immune system.[9] They not only cause cancer, but also fibromyalgia and reproductive problems.[10] It is important to find safe personal care and cleaning products, and to avoid fragrances unless they are pure essential oils. Store food in glass jars instead of plastic containers, and use paper lunch wrap, not plastic.

Toxins can also come through vaccinations and dental practices. Mercury is one of the most dangerous substances on the planet, and yet thimerosal is used as a carrier for many vaccinations. (You can guess what 'mer' stands for).

Amalgam fillings

Silver or amalgam dental fillings contain around 50% mercury, 35% silver and various other metals. Mercury is more toxic than lead, cadmium and even arsenic. Furthermore there is no known toxic threshold for mercury vapour, meaning that even the smallest amount of mercury vapour can be harmful. Mercury is continually released from amalgam fillings in the form of mercury vapour, and chewing, brushing and drinking hot liquid all increase this.

Scientific research has demonstrated that mercury, even in small amounts, can damage the brain, heart, lungs, liver, kidneys, thyroid gland, blood cells, enzymes, hormones, and as well, suppresses the body's immune system. Mercury has been shown to pass through the placental membrane in pregnant women, causing permanent damage to the brain of the developing foetus. Because cancer is a disease of toxicity, the mercury's contribution to the cause of cancer must be considered. Amalgam fillings were first used in Paris in 1832, and in that same year the world's first case of Multiple Sclerosis was reported. In a study involving the US FDA, out of 113 MS patients, 86 reported significant improvement or total cure at some time after the fillings were replaced.

Mercury is attracted to fat, so for detoxification, raw eggs in juice, with the addition of cold-pressed olive oil, vitamins C, E and antioxidants are recommended. The mercury will be eliminated as it clings to the ingested fats and passes through the body. People on juice fasts may experience severe detoxification effects, so may need to include some raw eggs and olive oil. Only a biological dentist, using special apparatus including a rubber oral dam and mask, should remove amalgam fillings. *11*

Radiation

We are becoming more and more surrounded by it – mobile phones, microwave ovens, and electrical fields, computers. Studies are now showing that these things can cause cancer.

Parasites

One of the principle causes in weakening an immune system is yeast and parasite infection. Yeast and parasites thrive on sugar, so that's another reason for eliminating sugar from the diet. Yeast, or candida, also thrives when our good intestinal flora is destroyed by drugs, such as antibiotics or chemotherapy. A good intestinal flora supplement, as well as a predominance of raw plant foods in the diet can help keep this under control. Once or twice a year it is wise to eliminate parasites from you system. There are herbal formulas to deal with parasites. These herbs include wormwood, black walnut, fennel, pau d'arco, cloves, slippery elm, and garlic. *12*

Stress

Stress lowers the body's efficiency to deal with free radicals and cancer may result. Stress is a major cause of many illnesses. The body cannot effectively fight the onslaught of disease if under stress. Inner peace and happiness on the other hand promote good health. The only way to obtain complete inner peace is by having a right relationship with the Creator, and as well, a right relationship with the people with whom our lives are linked. Problems and hurts from the past need to be dealt with. The ability to forgive others is the key to resolving bitterness. Freedom from stress and having a contented spirit is extremely important. A contented spirit, along with peace, harmony and happiness in the home, comes from trust in our Creator.

It is also important to express ourselves in fun and enjoyment. It is scientifically proven that joy and laughter produce chemicals (endorphins) in the body that encourage healing. Hence the old saying, 'laughter is the best medicine'. A change from the daily routine is good stress-therapy. This could be taking a restful holiday, reading a good book or taking a walk.

Preventing cancer

Living in fear of cancer will only add to the problem. The good news is that we don't have to fear cancer. Rather than waiting for the symptoms to appear, and then treat the symptoms, it is far better to prevent the disease in the first place. Taking steps to avoid illness is called preventative medicine, which involves learning to build up one's resistance and thereby lowering one's susceptibility to illness. Prevention comes through nutrition, exercise, avoidance of toxins and avoidance of stress. Build your immune system! It's much easier to prevent cancer, than to fight it once you've got it. The average person doesn't think about cancer until they get it.

We need to train our children in healthy living. After all, they will probably be growing up in a world that is more polluted than the present. They need to know how to safeguard their health through healthy living. Parents need to set an example by eating and buying the right foods, and involving children in the preparation of healthy food. Healthy living not only includes food, but also good vitamin and mineral supplementation, minimising toxic chemicals, exercising regularly and maintaining good spiritual and emotional health.

Endnotes

1. Virkler, M & P., *Go Natural*, U.S.A. 1995, p. 6
2. Van Straten, M., & Griggs, B., *Super Foods*, U.K., 1990, p. 30
3. *The Melbourne Age*, Aust., December 7, 1995
4. Caroll, K., *Experimental Evidence of Dietary Factors and Hormone Dependent Cancers*

5. Campbell, T.C, & Cox, C., *The China Project*, U.S.A., 1996
6. Ibid
7. Epstein, Samuel, *Unreasonable Risk*, U.S.A., 2002
8. Journal of American College of Toxicology; Vol. 2,1983
9. Woollams, C., *Oestrogen, the Killer in our Midst*, U.K., 2004, pp. 102-106
10. Hollingsworth, E., *Take Control of your Health*, 2002, Aust. p. 142
11. Martin, G., *Lifestyle Excellence*, Oct-Dec 2003, Aust
12. Woollams. op. cit., p. 97

chapter seven

DIET for CANCER patients

Paul's diet is based on recommendations from naturopaths and on principles from the Gerson diet. While every cancer patient needs a diet designed specifically for them by their own naturopath, there are basic principles that will be consistent for all cases of cancer. Please consult with your own health professionals before beginning a diet.

What is the Gerson Diet?

Max Gerson, born in Germany in 1881, was a medical doctor who used diet and other natural treatments to deal with cancer. For twenty years he treated hundreds of patients who had been given up to die. His success rate was 50%, which for his day was exceptional among alternative practitioners, and this percentage is far higher than current day orthodox treatments. He stated: "this percentage could be higher if there were better cooperation from the family physician, the patient himself and less resistance from the family against such a strict regime." [1]

Using a whole-body approach to healing, Gerson's therapy is based on the body's magnificent ability to heal itself, with no damaging side-effects. He believed that degenerative diseases were brought on by degraded food, water and air. Gerson therapy flooded the body with nutrients from organically grown fruits and vegetables. Oxygenation of the blood is usually more than doubled with the consumption of vast amounts of raw fruits and vegetables, and this in itself destroys cancer cells.

Max Gerson's therapy:
- Fresh juices, (raw carrot, apple and green-leaf), were consumed 13 times per day, (one glass every hour).
- Meals consisted of freshly prepared organically grown fruits, vegetables and wholegrains, and no animal protein.
- Coffee enemas were given for detoxification.
- Supplementation using natural substances was extremely important.

The aims of the diet for cancer patient

1. To eliminate toxins.
2. To use the natural healing properties of raw fruits and vegetables, herbs and minerals.
3. To maximise digestion so that what you eat works most effectively to improve your health.
4. To allow the body to heal itself.
5. To reduce the intake of high protein foods. High protein foods lead to an acidic system, whereas raw plant foods lead to an alkaline system. Cancer will not survive in an alkaline environment.

Elimination of toxins

Since cancer is a response to a build-up of toxins in the body, the first step is to eliminate them. Before beginning the diet, Paul attended a nine-day live-in session at Living Valley Springs, involving juice fasting, colonic irrigation and liver detoxification. For the first three days, vegetable juices were consumed, followed by two days of eating fruits and vegetables, then another three days of juice fasting.

Drinking large amounts of pure water first thing in the morning, and between meals is important as toxins continue to be eliminated. Drinking with meals reduces the efficiency of digestion. Drinks are taken 2 hours after completing a meal. Meals are taken 5 hours apart, with no snacking in between. The last meal is taken as early as 5 p.m. and no later than 6 p.m., so that there is no undigested food in the stomach while sleeping. The evening meal should be smaller than the midday meal.

Healing properties of raw fruits and vegetables

Plant foods contain many natural healing properties. Your food is your medicine. Fruit and vegetables are best if consumed fresh, vine-ripened and organically grown. Picking and eating straight from the garden is ideal, but of course not often possible. Growing your own parsley is a good idea. Five vegetables have particular value in fighting cancer. These are the cruciferous vegetables: broccoli, cabbage, asparagus, Brussels sprouts, and cauliflower. Carrots are good for betacarotene, another cancer fighter. Beetroot is also good for fighting cancer. These vegetables can be eaten raw or juiced. It may not always be possible to obtain organically grown fruit and vegetables. At times when you only have the choice of regular produce, choose fruits and vegetables that can be peeled or washed well. Celery, strawberries, broccoli and cauliflower absorb pesticides more easily because of their structure.

Maximising the efficiency of the digestive system

'Don't eat and drink at the same time' is a good rule to follow. Drink half an hour before a meal and two hours after.

Don't mix fruit and vegetables at the one meal. Eating both together interferes with good digestion. The tradition of eating fresh fruit after a meal is not a good one. Fruit digests quickly and wants to charge through the digestive system. Vegetables and starches take longer. Fruit is best eaten on an empty stomach, so that it can perform the cleansing job that it is meant to do. It makes an excellent breakfast, as it helps the body's natural elimination process at that time of day.

Juicing

Using a juicer can maximise the healing properties of these vegetables. Juicing removes the solids, releasing the phytochemicals from the fibre. This enables the body to assimilate the vital elements of the fruit and vegetables quickly, without any hindrance to the digestion, and without destroying any of the plant enzymes. Plant pulp and fibre take hours to digest, while juices may take only twenty minutes. Some people ask, "Why can't I just eat the fruits and vegetables without juicing them?" The reason is, to eat the amount required for healing would be impossible. *2*

Juices are excellent between meals because they allow the stomach to rest, while at the same time, absorbing massive amounts of nutrients. Juicing provides extra nutrients between meals, without starting up the digestive process again. An occasional juice fast is also an excellent way to energise and detoxify.

Use a high quality centrifuge or press juicer, available through health outlets and not through department stores. This type of juicer will maximise the amount of juice extracted and will not destroy the enzymes. It will also oxygenate the juice. A good combination for vegetable juice is carrot, beetroot and celery. To make half a glass of juice you would need about 4 medium carrots, a stick of celery and about ¼ of a medium sized beetroot. Adding some apple is also an option. (Mixing fruits and vegetables in juices will not undermine digestion because juices are taken on an empty stomach.) If you can't find organic celery, use leafy green vegetables, such as cabbage, spinach and parsley.

There are many testimonials to the healing power of juices alone. Rudolf Breuss, born in Austria in 1899, looked for alternative treatments for cancer, and discovered a book written 300 years before on the healing power of fruit and vegetable juices. Breuss maintained that cancer feeds and grows from proteins. He deduced that if one fasted, using juices and herbal teas to detoxify, cleanse and eliminate, the cancer would starve. Over 45,000 people testified that Breuss's simple treatment had cured them, often after they had been 'given up' by the orthodox medical establishment. *3*

Growing your own wheat grass
Wheat grass is an extremely nutritious ingredient to juice with your vegetables. It is easy to grow, and it grows extremely fast. Just take a plant pot with a saucer under-

neath. Fill the pot with good soil and set it up inside on your kitchen windowsill. Buy some organic wheat from a health shop. Sprinkle some wheat on top of the soil. Water daily. It should be ready to use in about a week. Cut a handful of wheat grass with scissors. Fold it in half and juice it with your carrots.

Allowing the body to heal itself

Given time, the body will heal itself if given the right ingredients. A cleansing program is the first step one must take. Herbs and nutrients all assist the body in its healing work. If the diet seems too difficult, remember that you are following it to save your life!

The Diet

Following the fasting-cleansing program, Paul maintained a strict diet for several months. The diet can be summarised as:
1. 80% raw fruit OR vegetables at every meal (not both).
2. 20% cooked plant food at every meal.
3. No meat, no dairy products, no sugar, no heat-extracted oils, no margarine.
4. No commercially processed food.
5. Pure water and vegetable juices only between meals.

It is important to maintain a strict diet in the early stages of nutritional therapy. Maintain the 80% raw food at every meal and no animal products, except for mercury-free fish oils. After a few months, add some free-range eggs.

Vitamin B17

Vitamin B17, also known as laetrile or amygdalin, has vital cancer fighting properties. It is naturally occurring in a variety of foods, such as buckwheat, berries, lentils, linseeds, almonds, cashews and millet, but it is most concentrated in the seeds of apricots, peaches, plums, nectarines and apples. It is a form of cyanic acid, toxic to cancer cells, although not toxic to other cells in the body. [4]

Pineapple, paw paw and additional pancreatic enzymes should be taken in the morning. The kernels should be taken throughout the day and not taken all at once. They should be chewed, or ground and then chewed. They can be added to foods to help disguise the bitter taste, e.g. with mashed banana. However they should be masticated, even if ground.

The Hunzas, renowned for longevity, were traditional growers of apricots. They cracked the seeds of apricots, ground the kernels and added them to their food.

Dr. Ernst Krebs junior, medical graduate of Illinois in 1941, with his father, researched the use of enzymes and vitamin B17, in their treatment of cancer. He built upon the research of Professor John Beard, from Edinburgh University, 30 years before. Krebs found that vitamin B17 was extremely toxic to cancer cells, although harmless to normal cells. He discovered that the cancer cell had a protein covering, and if the body's pancreatic enzymes dissolved that covering, then the cancer cell can be destroyed by the white blood cells, but even more effectively by vitamin B17. The two components, Hydrogen cyanide and especially Benzaldehyde in the B17, are extremely toxic to cancer cells. [5]

In normal cells, the enzyme rhodinase, produced in the liver, renders B17 harmless. Every day we produce several-hundred cancer cells. We need to destroy them early with a diet rich in B17. Vitamin B17 seeks out and destroys only the cancer cells. Krebs recommended eating ten apricot kernels per day for life as a preventive measure. A maximum of 5 kernels at any one time in a two-hour period is recommended to prevent excess B17 building up in the liver. Vitamin B17 should not be taken by people with liver cancer, or by people with liver malfunction. [6]

Dr Binzel, who uses nutritional therapy along with vitamin B17, explains that removing the tumour does not correct the defects in an individual's defence mechanism, so it is likely that the tumour will come back. Dr. Binzel does not start his patients on laetrile until the patients have been on vitamin and mineral supplements, enzymes and an anti-cancer diet for ten days to two weeks. He finds that laetrile seems to have little or no effect until a sufficient quantity of other vitamins and minerals are in the body.

Zinc, for example, is the transportation mechanism for the Laetrile. The body will not rebuild any tissue without sufficient vitamin C. [7]

FOODS TO AVOID

For those who have cancer, the following foods will reduce the body's ability to heal itself, so should be avoided. For those who wish to avoid cancer, then these foods should be eaten in moderation if at all.

Meat

In population studies, high meat intake has been associated with high incidence of cancer. Animal proteins are surplus to the body's needs and therefore impose a heavy tax on the organs during digestion. Red meat, in particular, causes acidity. If you have cancer then you need to give your body every possible chance to heal itself, so only eat simple foods that do not tax the digestive system.

Dairy products

These are high in fat and protein and create an acidic system.

Processed sugars

The molecules in refined sugar are too large for the body to break down. The result is a depressed immune system.

Salt

Avoid all refined salt and use only hand-harvested natural sea salt.

Food additives

These include artificial colourings, flavourings and preservatives that only add toxins to the body. Despite the fact that chemical additives are regarded as safe by food manufacturers, most chemicals are toxic in the long-term. The accumulation of toxins over time may cause allergies, cancer and other illnesses.

Tea and coffee

These contain caffeine and tannin, which deplete nutrient levels. Caffeine is an irritant to the kidneys, which lowers the efficiency of the body to eliminate toxins through urination. For cancer patients, an efficient elimination system is crucial. Caffeine also reduces the body's ability to absorb iron, and is a diuretic. This means that it causes dehydration.

Live yeast

Yeast, which remains active for 24 hours after baking, can cause fungal growth. Sour rye dough bread is a better option, but it is still better to keep bread to a minimum and eat brown rice instead.

Oils that have been heated

Oils become carcinogenic when heated and can become rancid when exposed to light. Even cold-pressed oils should not be kept too long and should be kept in a lightproof container. All commercial oils, unless labelled 'cold-pressed', have already been heated once. Margarine should definitely be avoided.

Baking powder

This includes food made with self-raising flour. Such rising agents inhibit digestion and reduced iron absorption.

Refined carbohydrates

These are the white flours, white sugar and white rice. They contain no fibre, little food value and slow down the digestive system causing inefficient elimination, a major cause of cancer.

Smoked, barbequed and burnt food

These contain carcinogenic substances (toxic). Never eat food that is burnt.

Alcohol
Most alcoholic beverages contain high sugar levels and chemical residue from the production process. Drinking alcohol adds a further load to your liver, requiring further detoxifying. *8*

Food cooked in microwave ovens
Food cooked, heated or defrosted in a microwave oven causes change in our blood. The blood, in its changed state shows symptoms of the initial stage of cancer. This was the finding of Swiss biologist Dr. Hans Ulrich-Hertel, upon studying the extreme dangers of microwave ovens in 1989. Hertel was the first scientist to carry out a quality study on the effects of microwaved nutrients on the blood and physiology of human beings. The results also proved for the first time that microwave energy (retained in food) which promotes cancer, could actually be transmitted to humans through food, and not just by being near the microwave itself. The latter has long been known. Microwaved food is commonly served in hotels and restaurants. *9*

Other studies supporting the carcinogenic effects of microwaves:
• A 1984 study by the University of Washington indicated a carcinogenic effect in animal tests.
• Australian expert, Dr. John Holt, with 25 years of research on this issue, has found that a 5 minute burst of microwave radiation can stimulate a cancer to grow 100 times faster for half an hour.
• Russian tests on microwaved food found carcinogens in virtually all foods tested. These included meats, milk, cereals, frozen and raw fruits and vegetables.

What are the effects of microwaved food?
The Russian studies found the following:
• Higher percentage of cancerous cells in the blood
• Malfunctions in the lymphatic system, causing degeneration of the immune system.
• Higher incidence of stomach and intestinal cancers

Other problems:
- Some food cooks unevenly, meaning that the food may be cooked on the outside but raw on the inside.
- Hot spots and cold spots mean that some bacteria in the food will survive in the cold spots.
- Any food containing vegetable oil will become particularly carcinogenic due to the high heat.
- All microwave ovens leak toxic radiation while in operation, causing many health problems.
- Microwave radiation alters the substances it heats.
- Microwaved food is commonly served in hotels and restaurants, so eating out may not always be safe.

FOODS TO EAT

80% raw fruits or vegetables at every meal. The other 20% of the meal is made up from the following:

Whole grains
Brown rice, millet, buckwheat, quinoa

Lentils
Red, green or brown are suitable. Brown lentils are a more mature form of green lentils.

Dried beans & peas
Red kidney beans, haricot beans, lima beans, chick peas, split peas

Dried seaweed
Arame, boiled for 15 minutes and added to seasoned rice.

Cooked potatoes; sweet potatoes; pumpkin
Sweet potatoes are high in betacarotene.

Oats
These should be whole oats, and not the refined type.

Nuts and seeds
Almonds are especially good. They have anti-cancer properties. Ground flaxseeds are also good. Almonds, sunflower seeds and flaxseeds can be ground together in a coffee grinder.

Flaxseeds
Take a dessertspoon of flaxseeds and grind together with nuts, sunflower seeds and pepitas. Flaxseeds contain omega-3, omega-6 and vitamin B17.

Apricot kernels
No more than five kernels every two hours

Simple sugars
Use only honey or fruit concentrate as sweeteners. These do not depress the immune system. Use in moderation.

Unrefined salts
Use only hand-harvested unrefined sea salt.

THE DAILY ROUTINE
This is an example of a day's nutritional intake, including food supplements.

On rising
- 2 glasses warm water with lemon juice
- 2 teasp. liquid minerals
- Essiac tea and Special Herbal Tea

30 minutes later
- Glass of organic grape juice mixed with the following:
- 2 teasp. green barley powder
- 1 teasp. spirulina powder
- 1 teasp. vitamin C powder
- Noni juice or aloe vera juice
- Wait another 15 minutes before eating breakfast

Breakfast
- Large bowl of fresh fruit, including paw paw and pineapple
- 1 dessertsp. each of ground sunflower seeds, linseeds, almonds and pepitas, mixed with a little organic grape juice for a moist consistency.
- Antioxidant supplement e.g. pine bark and grape seed, or bee pollen
- Vitamin supplement

Mid morning
- Plenty of pure water (3 glasses or more)
- Vegetable juice (beetroot, carrot, celery, greens)

Lunch
- Fresh raw salad, including carrot, cabbage, raw beetroot, tomato, raw asparagus, broccoli, sprouts and plenty of greens.
- 20% cooked food. E.g. brown rice, cooked haricot beans in home-made sauce
- Vitamin supplement

Mid afternoon
- Plenty of pure water (3 glasses or more)

- Essiac tea, Special Herbal Tea
- Vegetable juice (beetroot, carrot, celery, greens) with the addition of green barley/spirulina powder

Evening meal
A smaller meal than lunch
- Raw vegetables plus any foods in the 20% cooked plant food category, e.g. legumes
- Vitamin supplement

Before bed
- Antioxidant supplement.

Essiac Tea
This is a traditional Canadian Indian remedy, known by three names: Essiac tea, Cassie Tea and Sheep Sorrel tea. The formula consists of cut burdock root (577 g), powdered sheep's sorrel leaves and stems (322 g), Turkish rhubarb (20 g) and powdered slippery elm bark (80.5 g). Mix loose herbs together to make a large quantity of tea. Store in an airtight container. Prepare the drink by taking ½ cup loose herb mixture and add to 1 litre of boiling water. Boil on the stove for 10 minutes. Cool, strain and pour into a glass jar. This will keep in the fridge for 3 days. Drink little and often throughout the day, e.g. 30 ml. 6 times a day. Add a little hot water to each drink.

Another tea that has similar anti-cancer properties is Jason Winter's tea.

Special Herbal Tea
Ask a naturopath to prescribe some loose herbs, specific to your needs, and make as a tea. This was the formula recommended for Paul by Living Valley Springs:

Clivers (60 g); Chaparral (40 g); Gotu Kola (50 g); Red Clover (60 g); Small-flowered willow (60 g)

This makes a large supply of loose tea. Store in airtight container and prepare daily as follows:
• Make the drink in a small teapot using one dessertspoon of herbs.
• Pour on approx. 1-cup boiling water and allow the tea to brew for a minimum of 20 minutes.

The tea does not have to be taken hot. It tastes better if taken cold. Take two drinks per day, on rising and mid-afternoon.

Some other useful herbs
• Herb for building the immune system: astragalus
• Herbs for the lymphatic system: poke root, burdoc and queen's delight
• Herbs for fighting cancer: red clover; mistletoe; violet leaves
• Herbs with excellent healing properties: withania, suma, St. Mary's thistle, bacopa, schisandra
• Herb for stimulating the circulatory system and enhancing the effectiveness of other herbs: Ginger
• Anti-cancer herb: turmeric (can be added to food)

Some cancer-fighting supplements
These are additional to mineral and vitamin supplements:
• Vitamin B17, found in apricot kernels
• Aloe vera (polysaccharides for cell-to-cell communication and building immune system)
• Noni juice (polysaccharides; regulates function of organs)
• Garlic (antioxidant and anti-parasite)
• Betacarotene (present in spirulina and orange vegetables)
• Grape seed extract (antioxidant)
• Pinus stobus (antioxidant from French Maritime Pine bark. Also called Pycnogenol).
• Ginko biloba
•Maiitake mushroom
• Ginseng

Oxygen therapy and exercise

Oxygen acts like an antioxidant, and helps reduce cancer cells. Paul received ozone therapy, where oxygen and ozone were administered by means of a sauna tent, oxygen being absorbed through the skin. There are various forms of oxygen therapy available. Drinking oxygenated water is also beneficial.

Exercise will also oxygenate the cells, as the lungs fill with fresh air and expel the stale air. Exercise gets the lymph moving. You must move the lymph daily to remove toxins from the cells. Jumping on a mini-trampoline daily, with emphasis on heels moving up and down but toes remaining in contact with the trampoline base, will stimulate lymph movement.

How long should I maintain a strict diet?

Max Gerson advised adhering to a total plant-food diet for about 4 months. The reason for a low calorie diet in the first 3 to 6 months after the initial cleanse is to allow the body to do the work of eradicating the cancer, and to prevent any overloading of the digestive system.

Paul began the diet in January 1997, following the 9-day cleansing and fasting therapy. A predominantly plant-based diet, with emphasis on raw, has now become a lifestyle. Paul maintained the 80% raw food diet, with no meat or dairy products for the first 6 months. Then he added some free-range eggs, a small amount of wild salmon and a slightly higher percentage of cooked food.

The practice of juicing and drinking pure water between meals should continue be part of the daily routine, as this is vital to the on-going healing process. Once you've had cancer, you must be serious about prevention for the rest of your life, even if the doctor tells you that you are 'in remission', or 'clear' of cancer. Vitamin, mineral and herbal supplements play a huge role in prevention – a lifetime commitment!

Many people ask initially, "Do I always have to eat salad?" It can be difficult in the winter to eat salad all the time. It is important to include some salad at every meal, but you can also eat hot raw vegetables in the winter. They can be prepared as a stir-fry, or just chopped finely and added to hot rice. They can also be stirred into hot soup, e.g. pumpkin, tomato, pea or bean soups. Serve freshly picked raw parsley with every vegetable meal. You soon acquire a taste for a plant-based diet, and you will be surprised how satisfying it is.

Even though Paul's physical examination indicated no sign of cancer, the new way of eating will be on-going for the rest of his life. This healthy diet has become a lifestyle for the whole family.

Other factors to consider in fighting cancer or avoiding it:
1. Plenty of sleep especially during hours of natural darkness
2. Peace of mind and no stress
3. Maintaining good emotional health
4. Times of relaxation
5. A relationship with the Creator
6. Putting aside past hurts and showing forgiveness towards others
7. Happiness and laughter (release chemicals in the body called endorphin)
8. Clean water (use a water filter)
9. Clean air
10. Exposure to sunlight for vitamin D
11. No harmful chemicals. Chemicals can be absorbed through skin into bloodstream. Use shampoo, toothpaste and other personal care products with safe ingredients. Avoid Sodium Lauryl Sulphate, Propylene Glycol, any chemical listed with a capital E. (e.g. DEA, TEA, PEG).
12. Avoid pesticides and chemical cleaning products.
13. Eat in moderation, even healthy foods.
14. No toxic substances into the body
15. Remove amalgam fillings in teeth. They leach mercury and other heavy metals into the body.
16. Hot and cold showering. Changing the shower temperature from hot to cold in

repetitive bursts, increases the flow of the lymph system and strengthens the immune system.

17. Regular exercise, especially jumping on a small round trampoline to get the lymph flowing. There are also special exercise machines available for stimulating lymph flow.

Endnotes

1. Gerson, M., *A Cancer Therapy – Results of Fifty Cases and The Cure of Advanced Cancer by Diet Therapy*, 5th edition, p. 33
2. Cilento, R., *Heal Cancer: Choose you own survival path*, Aust., 1993 p. 59
3. Breuss, Rudolph, & Hemmes, Hilde, Cancer/Leukemia, Austria
4. Binzel, P., *Alive and Well*, U.S.A.,1994, p. 23-24
5. Woollams. C., *The Tree of Life*, 2004, p. 151
6. Binzel, P., op cit, p 24
7. Binzel, P., op.cit., pp. 25 & 99
8. Cilento, R., op.cit., p. 42
9. *Microwave ovens – A Recipe for Cancer*, The Consumer Association of Penang, p. 4-5

chapter eight

food SUPPLEMENTS for EVERYONE

Do we really need food supplements?

Dr. Max Gerson states: "The damage that modern civilisation brings into our lives begins with the soil, where artificial fertilisation leads to the displacement of mineral content, and changes the flora of microbes combined with the exodus of the earth-worms." [1]

Dr. Gerson's book entitled A Cancer Therapy gives the results of tests, which show what happens to the soil when it is cropped year after year and not allowed to lie fallow every seventh year. [2]

A wealth of clinical experience has validated the use of vitamins, minerals and herbs in fighting cancer. For example, the Hoxsey Biomedical Clinic in Tijuana, Mexico, is a mecca for cancer sufferers from across the U.S. border. Physicians, such as Dr. Paavo Arriolo are in the forefront of developing successful treatments.

Many people think that the taking of supplements is wrong, and that we should get all our nutritional needs from the food we eat. However, in this day and age, it may not be possible. Supplements are not only beneficial in the healing of cancer, but in the healing of many illnesses. Even healthy people should take nutritional supplements, as a preventative measure for avoiding illness.

The following list of supplements has been recommended in the treatment of cancer, but of course they are also beneficial for maintenance of general health. Before buying vitamin or mineral tablets it is important to be assured of their quality. Reputable nutritionists express concern about the pharmaceutical standards in manufacturing of supplements. Many lack the purity and potency specified on the label. Also, many pass through the intestinal system before they can be broken down. Most are made from synthetic (as opposed to natural) substances, which cannot be properly assimilated by the body.

Laboratory research has shown that nutrients can be ineffective if consumed in the wrong amounts. Many work together, but some can actually prevent our bodies from making full use of the others. Therefore a truly balanced nutritional program is essential. High scientific standards are essential in producing effective nutritional supplements. Low-cost supplements are inferior and of little use. If you really value your health, use only high-quality supplements.

Micro minerals

Humans are designed to derive minerals from plant sources and not inorganic rock sources. Microorganisms in the soil convert inorganic minerals into a form that is useable by plants. The human body easily utilises minerals in this form. The most bio-available minerals are liquid, colloidal, plant based minerals. It is possible to absorb 98% of the minerals in a good colloidal mineral formula. However we would absorb only about 5% of an inorganic mineral supplement, so these are really a waste of money. [3]

Because the soils are so depleted of minerals therefore making plants depleted, mineral supplementation is essential for everyone who wants to avoid metabolic disease. There are approximately 66 trace minerals essential to good health. They are called trace minerals because they are only needed in very small amounts, but they are catalysts for various chemical reactions that need to occur within the body. Trace minerals include iron, zinc, copper, iodine, chromium, manganese and selenium. They should not be taken separately, but in a balanced colloidal formula. Selenium is particularly important in protecting against cancer, and it is known to increase the effects of vitamin E. It is also an antioxidant. Zinc is also worth a mention. A deficiency in zinc would severely impair the body's defences against cancer.

Macro minerals

These are the minerals essential to health, required in larger amounts. They play important roles in maintaining body functions. Macro minerals include calcium, potassium, phosphorus and magnesium. Max Gerson believed that cancer may arise in a body that is deficient in potassium, as a result of too high a sodium diet. Potassium is necessary in the maintenance of normal metabolism, regulation and production of hormones, enzymes and co-enzymes.

Antioxidants

Grape seed extract and White Pine Bark, (also called pycnogenol), are very powerful antioxidants. In 1534 the French explorer, Jacques Cartier, was stranded on the St. Lawrence River in Canada for the winter. With most of his crew dying or very ill, Cartier met an Indian who showed him how to make a tea from white pine-bark, which the local people believed had remarkable properties. Four hundred years later, Professor Jacques Masquelier read of this expedition and initiated research to isolate the ingredients found in the tea made from the white pine bark. During his research he also found similar ingredients in other botanicals, most notably in the seeds and skins of red grapes, which were similar in composition to the pine-bark extract. They were both found to be outstanding antioxidants. Antioxidants are our body's defence system against free radicals. [4]

Pycnogenol has been shown in clinical studies to be 25 times more effective that vitamin C and 50 times more effective than vitamin E as an antioxidant. In fact, pycnogenol appears to be the most powerful antioxidant ever discovered. It is an anti-inflammatory, antihistamine, strengthens blood vessels, acts against bleeding gums and much more. Pycnogenol could be described as a 'super-smart missile' that targets any damaged cells, restoring them. Pycnogenol is not only recommended for those with cancer, but also as a preventative measure. [5]

VITAMINS

It is essential to take vitamins, in a totally balanced formula. The problem with some inferior supplements is that they may not be in appropriate combinations. Large doses of one vitamin may decrease the absorption of another. The formula must be high quality, with ingredients that work synergistically.

A particular combination of natural vitamins has been discovered to dramatically improve heart health, but at the same time help people with cancer because of its role in detoxification. This formula is used by doctors, administered intravenously, and known as chelation therapy.

Chelation therapy has been used for many years, particularly in Europe. The formula attracts and binds heavy metals, and extracts them from the body tissues so they can be released for excretion by the kidneys. Lead for example, is stored in all body tissues, including blood, bones and brain. [6]

It is possible to obtain an oral chelation formula. This formula is very effective, and is far easier to administer than the intravenous formula. Oral chelated vitamin tablets ensure bioavailability, and help to detoxify. This is particularly important for people with toxic overload.

It is extremely beneficial for people who need to detoxify. This may include cancer patients or children with Attention Deficit Disorder. Eve Hillary, who suffered from chemical toxicity, and whose son developed A.D.D for the same reasons, found chelation therapy to be a vital tool for recovery.

Vitamin C

For those with cancer, additional ascorbic acid is important. Vitamin C can effectively neutralise or minimise the damaging effect of most chemical carcinogens (toxins) in food and the environment. [7]

Vitamin C increases the production of antibodies, increases the efficiency of the immune system and protects against infection. It is also an antioxidant and protects against free radicals. It is anti-stress and aids the absorption of iron. The richest food sources of vitamin C are blackcurrants, strawberries, citrus fruits, green peppers, raw cabbage, spinach and parsley.

Vitamin E

This is an antioxidant, which increases the oxygenation of cells, which is of crucial importance in the prevention of cancer. The richest food sources of vitamin E are: extra-virgin olive oil, nuts, sunflower seeds, whole grains, dark green vegetables and eggs. [8]

Betacarotene

Vitamin A, and betacarotene in particular, are potent antioxidants. They combat free-radical activity and are vital to the integrity of cell membranes and the body's immune system. The best food sources are the dark green, yellow and orange fruits and vegetables, particularly mature carrots. Large quantities of betacarotene are also present in spirulina . Vitamin A protects against cancer development in the epithelial tissues, which are sites where cancer usually starts. [9]

The juicing of fresh organic carrots, with the addition of beetroot and celery, and some green spirulina/barley leaf powder, twice daily, will help supply the extra need for vitamin A and betacarotene.

Polysaccharides

When errors occur in the way cells send signals from one to the other, cancer can occur. Healthy signaling and message flow is largely dependent on polysaccharides. A number of naturally occurring substances have been identified as having high polysaccharide content. These are the medicinal mushrooms, reishi, shitake, maii-take, cordyceps and oyster mushrooms. Aloe vera and noni juice are both excellent supplements for optimal functioning of cells and therefore very beneficial to those with cancer. The sugars of fruits and vegetables such as carrots, leeks, radishes, apples, pears, tomatoes, corn, garlic, and citrus fruits also contain polysaccharides. *10*

Spirulina

This microscopic blue-green algae is found in the alkaline waters of shallow lakes. Spirulina is known as a 'wonder food', and was part of the staple diet of the ancient Aztec civilisation. It is high in protein and iron. It also contains liberal quantities of betacarotene, chlorophyll, vitamin E and the minerals phosphorus, potassium, calcium, magnesium and zinc. *11*

Green barley

Green Barley is rich in vitamins, minerals, amino acids, chlorophyll and live enzymes. When taken with liquid, this richly nutritious food is quickly absorbed and utilised for detoxification and regeneration. *12*

Shark's Cartilage and Bovine Cartilage

Shark's cartilage is now established by extensive long-term quantitative and clinical research as a therapeutic food. Cartilage in the diet, (approx. 9 gm. per day), or topically applied, has been shown to heal intractable wounds; to be anti-inflammatory; to be analgesic in arthritic and cancer pain; to stop tumour growth; to restore movement and boost immune function. Quality bovine cartilage, (from beef), is also effective.*13*

The information on supplements, presented in this chapter, is an introduction for one's further research. The information is not to be considered as medical advice and anyone wishing to treat an existing condition is advised to seek the help of a reputable health care professional, informed in the area of natural therapy.

Endnotes

1. Cited in Virkler, M. & P., *Go Natural*, USA ,1991, p. 64
2. Ibid.
3. *Colloidal Minerals, Sparks of Life*, USA, 1998
4. Arriola, Paavo, M.D., Hoxsey Biomedical Clinic, Tijuana, Mexico
5. Virkler, M. & P., *Go Natural*, p. 125
6. Hillary, Eve, *Children of a Toxic Harvest*, Aust., 1999, p.147
7. Troll, Walter, M.D, *Professor of Environmental Medicine*, N.Y.
8. *Underwater Treasures*: leaflet published by Natural Facts.
9. Arriola, Paavo, M.D., op cit.
10. Woollams, C., *The Tree of Life*, U.K., 2004, pp. 150-151
11. Cilento, Ruth, *Heal Cancer; Choose Your own Survival Path*, Aust., 1993, pp. 146-147
12. Silver Cord Magazine, May 1997.
13. *The MediFood Report*, October 1996

chapter nine

DEADLY lifestyle DISEASES

What are the leading causes of death today? Contagious disease is no longer the threat that it once was. Today our Western society is plagued with the killers of affluence. These are called metabolic diseases or degenerative diseases because they are not caught. Six of these deadly diseases are: heart disease, stroke, cancer, excess weight, diabetes and osteoporosis.

These diseases creep up on people as their bodies fail to perform their proper functions. Putting the wrong fuel in the car will eventually cause serious problems. Putting the wrong fuel in our bodies will do the same. As well as looking at the whole host of 'bad' things one can put into the body, we need to look at what is not being put in. Not having enough minerals can cause a break down of the immune system and health degeneration. We need to be putting the good nutrients in.

The stresses of modern living bombard our bodies with more toxins than ever. Toxins appear in cleaning products, personal care items, perfumes, printing dyes, inks, paints, carpets and upholstery.
We may be surrounded by toxicity and stress, but don't give up. We can do something about it! By taking these preventative measures we can avoid the deadly lifestyle

diseases and have quality of life in old age. Here are some preventative steps you can take:

1. Eat mostly plant foods.
2. Avoid processed food as much as possible.
3. Drink plenty of water.
4. Supplement with minerals, vitamins and antioxidants.
5. Get rid of toxins in your home, including toxins in personal care items.
6. Allow time for relaxation and find peace of mind.

HEART DISEASE

Heart disease is the leading cause of death in the western world today. Improper diet causes sludge, called plaque, slowly clogging the arteries until blood can no longer flow to deliver vital oxygen and nutrients to your heart muscles. This causes a heart attack. *1*

The government is spending millions on research, medication and bi-pass surgery, and yet the research has already been done. Heart disease is preventable. How do we prevent heart disease? Three factors are important: diet, exercise and supplementation. The same three steps apply if you have the condition.

DIET

Don't necessarily be guided by foods that receive 'the heart health tick'. Do avoid saturated fat, found in meat and dairy products, and especially avoid refined processed oils, like cooking oils and margarine. These can be more dangerous than saturated fat.

Take on the 'Diet for cancer patients' and drink plenty of water.

EXERCISE

Avoid stress and do adequate regular exercise.

SUPPLEMENTS

One of the most amazing developments in the prevention and treatment of heart conditions is chelation therapy. This is a special nutritional formula, given intravenously or in tablet form, that has no side-effects. Chelation means 'to claw'. This very powerful nutritional formula, when introduced into the body, claws and removes blockages to arteries, restoring blood flow.

Numerous double-blind studies have shown the success of chelation therapy. There is an 85-90% collective success rate. One study carried out in New Zealand, showed that 85% of the participants, scheduled for bi-pass surgery, no longer needed surgery after 6 months on chelation therapy. However in most countries, conventional medicine has rejected this therapy because money and politics have taken the place of a concern for health. (Bi-pass surgery brings in millions of dollars each year.) The problem with bi-pass surgery is that after 5 years, the plaquing starts all over again. [2]

Dr. Bill Davidson, who has developed a very good oral chelation formula, explains how oral chelation therapy works. Let's look at the arteries and veins. Arteries carry oxygen to the cells. The veins carry carbon dioxide from the cells back to the lungs. The arteries have an extra layer of muscle. Problems occur more readily in the arteries than the veins because of the hardening of this extra layer of muscle – a bit like a garden hose lying in the sun. It lacks flexibility and may crack. When arteries lose their flexibility they do not expand as they should. The pressure builds up and the heart has to work much harder to pump blood through the arteries. Damage occurs easily. Hardening is caused by free-radicals. Calcium and cholesterol can collect at the site of the damage. This reduces the diameter of the artery leading to reduction in blood flow.

When there is an abrasion in the arterial wall, plaque may go to this point in an attempt to repair the damage. This attempt to repair causes a build-up of plaque, which in turn leads to arterial blockage. Chelation therapy gently claws away and gradually removes the build-up of plaque on the arterial wall, at the same time repairing the damage.

As chelation therapy repairs damage to artery walls, it can also repair any cell in your body. It not only helps the cardio-vascular system, but can assist with any cell damage. While chelation therapy is most beneficial for heart health and prevention of stroke, Dr. Davidson explains that it is also extremely beneficial as a preventative or healing agent for arthritis and cancer. [3]

STROKE

Strokes are caused by the same problem that causes heart attack. The arteries of the brain harden and clog up, eventually shutting off the flow of blood to vital parts of the brain. [4]

A stroke is the secondary effect of a heart or circulatory condition. There are two kinds of stroke:
1. When the blood supply is prevented by clotting, (thrombosis).
2. When a haemorrhage results form a ruptured artery wall and consequently loss of supply to the brain. [5]

To prevent stroke, take on the same three steps as for heart disease, and if you have ever experienced a stroke, then these steps are absolutely necessary.

EXCESS WEIGHT

You may be saying that this is not a disease. That's true, but if you are overweight, your chances of contracting a metabolic disease are very high. One study showed that overweight people had 40% more risk of getting cancer. By contrast, smoking 'only' increased the risk by 25%. There is also a clear link between excess weight and heart disease. Overweight people also have more hormone imbalances because of extra amounts of hormones trapped in their fat. The hormones stored within the fat can reach dangerous levels. [6]

Weight Loss through lifestyle - the only way

What do you look for in a sound weight loss plan? To begin with, let's not focus on the word 'diet', because a diet makes us think of a severe cut back in food rations for a limited period of time. This is not what we're looking at in effective weight loss. We are not talking about starving ourselves or depriving ourselves. We are talking about making some positive radical changes to a lifestyle where the best food can be enjoyed at every meal.

There are three basic things to look for if you are serious about losing weight:
1. Taking control of the type of food you eat.
2. Regular exercise – at least 60 minutes per day.
3. Acknowledgement that a life-long change in habits is required.

Some interesting statistics:
Only about 5% of people who follow commercial diet programs actually lose weight and remain close to that weight. For most, one-third of the weight lost during dieting is regained within one year after the person stops the program. Almost all the weight is regained after five years. [7]

Every person who wants to lose weight has to look at a new way of eating. They must choose an eating plan that minimises hunger and fatigue, but at the same time is low in calories. It is important to be patient about losing weight, expecting to lose no more than half a kilo per week. Losing weight too quickly creates a yo-yo effect, and soon those kilos will be back where they came from. [8]

What is the best food for weight loss?
There are many 'diets' that claim inevitable weight loss, but really the best way to stay trim and healthy is to eat unprocessed foods. Now on first hearing this may sound radical, and even boring, but that's because we have lost the ability to appreciate the delicious flavours of natural food. The taste buds however can be trained. Have you ever heard of an 'acquired taste'? The more often you eat it, the more you will learn to enjoy it.

Raw plant food is the best food. It is full of nutrients and living enzymes. With most salad vegetables you can eat as much as you like and you won't put on weight. Aim to eat at least 50% raw plant food at every meal.

Breakfast should consist of fresh fruit, because this is the time of day when your body wants to eliminate waste, and enzymes in the fruit will help this process, and maintain good colon health. It's best not to include banana at this time of day. You can include some protein in the form of nuts and seeds – ground linseeds (flaxseeds), sunflower seeds and a few almonds are excellent.

Lunch and dinner should consist of at least 50% raw vegetables, a few steamed vegetables if you like, and some legumes such as dried beans, chickpeas or lentils. Legumes combine both protein and carbohydrates and are very nutritious. The occasional free-range egg is also beneficial.

Choose whole-food carbohydrates, such as sweet potato and brown rice. Avoid refined processed carbohydrates, such as white rice, bread, pasta and pastries. Keep in mind that raw salad should fill most of your plate. For an occasional sweet treat, a homemade oatmeal slice is a good one.

Drink plenty of pure water between meals. You will gradually learn to enjoy it. Herbal tea is also suitable. The aim is to cut out all foods that promote toxicity. Tea and coffee of course are in this category. A toxic body will produce more and more fat cells as needed, to store the toxic chemicals it absorbs. An effective antioxidant supplement will help with detoxifying. One containing grape seed extract and Maritime Pine-Bark is excellent.

You will need to find a good colloidal mineral supplement to prevent cravings. A deficiency in iron in particular can result in cravings. How do you know if you're mineral deficient? Unless you take a plant mineral supplement you can assume that you are low in essential minerals. The minerals are no longer in the soil, and therefore no longer in the plants.

A lifestyle – not a diet

Key points for a healthy weight-loss plan:

1. Eat unprocessed foods.
2. Major on raw fruits and vegetables – at least 50% of every meal
3. Eat fruit in the morning, on an empty stomach, or eat it alone as a snack when you are hungry, but not following a meal.
4. Replace meat with legumes, nuts in moderation, seeds and free-range eggs.
5. Cut out dairy products.
6. Drink plenty of pure water between meals. (Cut out regular tea and coffee.)
7. Take high quality mineral and antioxidant supplements.
8. Keep experimenting with new foods and new recipes, until you have found some healthy food that you really enjoy. Don't go hungry.
9. Know that you are loved. God created you. You're special. If you respect yourself, you will value yourself.

DIABETES

There are two types of diabetes:

Type 1

This often begins in late childhood, but can occur at any age. This is the rarer form, (10% of all diabetics) but also the more dangerous form. The pancreas loses its ability to synthesise insulin, so insulin injections must be given. [9]

Type 2

This is late-onset diabetes. The problem initially is not with the pancreas, but with the insulin receptors on the cell surfaces of certain body tissues, especially muscle tissue. The pancreas must work hard to increase insulin output to compensate, and eventually pancreatic function can fail. [10]

Type 2 diabetes seems to be brought on exclusively by our modern diet. In the past, it has been seen typically among people over 50, but today more and more adolescents and children are succumbing to it. A Harvard University study in 1997, on women, concluded that the ones who developed diabetes most commonly ate a low fibre diet, which was also high in refined sugars. A second study that year, on men, confirmed this. The study also found that hydrogenated vegetable oils could bring on diabetes. These are commonly found in fast foods and processed foods. Snack food is rich in sugar and hydrogenated oil. Fizzy drinks may contain 10 spoonfuls of sugar. Then consider breakfast cereal, biscuits, cakes and pasta. Yes, refined flour turns to sugar in our bodies. Refined pasta is no longer a living food. It has lost 80% of its vitamins, 90% of its minerals, and 100% of its fibre. [11]

One of the myths associated with diabetic diets, is that carbohydrate is bad. This is not correct. We need carbohydrate to fuel our muscles, red blood cells and brain. It is the type of carbohydrate that must be taken into account. If people don't eat carbohydrates, then they will eat fat and/or protein as a replacement. This is a recipe for a heart attack. The ranking of foods according to the effect it has on blood-sugar levels is called the 'glycemic index'. This is a dietary tool devised originally for people with diabetes, but it is also useful for weight loss. A food with a low glycemic index would score under 55. A food with a high glycemic index would get a score of above 70. High GI foods burn quickly and cause swings in the blood sugar levels. Low GI foods burn slowly and keep you going for longer. [12]

Just because a food has a low GI doesn't automatically make it good for you. You also need to take into account the quality of the food in terms of fat, protein, vitamin and mineral content and purity, as outlined in chapter 3. For example, meat may have a low glycemic index, but may contain too much fat and protein. In general, unprocessed foods have a low glycemic index, while refined processed foods have a high glycemic index. Don't forget to take into account the amount of food you are eating. Over eating in general can cause a rise in blood sugar.

Examples of low GI foods:

Meat	0
Lettuce	10
Pecan nuts	10

Green vegetables	15
Carrots, raw	20
Grapefruit	25
Kidney beans	27
Chick peas	28
Apricots, (dried)	30
Lentils, (cooked)	30
Milk	31
Pear, (fresh)	38
Apple, (raw)	38
Peach, (fresh)	40
Carrots, (cooked)	41
Spaghetti	41
Orange	44
Sweet potato	44
Oats	49
Buckwheat, (cooked)	54
Banana, (not very ripe)	52

Examples of moderate GI foods

Banana, (ripe)	55
Brown rice	55
Sweet corn	55
Rice, (basmati white)	58

Examples of high GI foods

Raisins	64
Potatoes, (boiled)	62
Coca-cola	63
Wholemeal bread	71
Rice, (white Jasmine)	72
Honey	73

Refined breakfast cereals   75
Jelly beans   80

Summary

1. Don't eat big meals that cause insulin surges.
2. Don't eat any refined carbohydrate.
3. Drink water.
4. Eat raw fruit and vegetables, cooked pulses, nuts, brown rice, buckwheat and sweet potatoes.
5. Exercise one hour per day.

Osteoporosis

Dairy products, despite popular opinion, are not the answer to osteoporosis. In the Western world we consume the highest volumes of dairy products in the world, and have the highest blood calcium levels, but the lowest bone calcium levels. The high level of protein in milk causes calcium to be actually drawn out of the bones, in an attempt to neutralise the acidity caused by high consumption of animal products.

The milk fats are likely to bring with them all manner of hormones, antibiotics, toxins, pesticides and herbicides. Organic milk, which may be free of these problems, still creates acidity and causes a problem with human digestion. High levels of fat and protein prevent absorption of zinc and calcium and depress magnesium and potassium levels. [13]

Osteoporosis is not simply caused by low calcium, but by low magnesium and poor vitamin D, toxins like steroids and excessive caffeine and sodium. Without magnesium you cannot absorb calcium into your cellular tissues or bones. Magnesium is needed for vitamin D synthesis. Low vitamin D levels mean low calcium absorption.

Best magnesium foods: nuts, pulses, mango, sweet corn, jacket potato, bananas, green leafy vegetables, millet, oats, buckwheat, brown rice.
Best calcium foods: green leafy vegetables, almonds, broccoli, dried beans, millet,

oats, buckwheat and brown rice.
Best vitamin D sources: mercury-free fish oil, sunshine

Magnesium levels lowered by: refined foods, stress, tea, coffee, alcohol, sugar, high carbohydrate and fat diets, which are empty of any nutritients.
Calcium levels are lowered by: soft drinks, tea and coffee, sugar, dairy products and refined foods. *14*

Osteoporosis is also caused by hormonal imbalance. It is scientifically linked to low progesterone and high oestrogen levels. Oestrogen dominance causes loss of bone density from ages 30-35 onwards. Oestrogen wears away the bones whereas progesterone builds them up. Today, nearly everyone is oestrogen dominant due to the fact that many mimic oestrogens surround us. An answer to this problem is to use wild yam cream, which the body absorbs and restores hormonal balance.

Other factors to consider for healthy bones are: weight bearing exercise —walking, climbing stairs, digging, aerobic exercises using weights
—and supplementation of other minerals and vitamins that are essential for the absorption of calcium.

Endnotes

1. Allen, R.G. *Your Health is in Danger*, p. 4
2. Dr. Rockford McCord, *Who Has Your heart?* (audio)
3. Dr. Bill Davidson, *Oral Chelation Therapy*, (audio)
4. Allen, R.G., op. cit.
5. Day, P., *The A.B.C.'s of Disease*, Credence, U.K., 2003, p. 223
6. Woollams, C., *The Tree of Life*, U.K., 2004, p.p. 109-110
7. Wardlaw, Hampl & DiSilvestro, *Perspectives in Nutrition,* 6th edition, U.S.A. 2004, p. 476
8. Ibid p. 477
9. Ibid p. 173

10. Ibid., p. 175
11. Woollams, C., op.cit., pp. 73–75
12. Brand-Miller, J., *The New Glucose Revolution*, Aust, 2003
13. Woollams, C., op. cit., p. 36
14. Ibid., pp. 26-27

chapter ten

MADE to be HEALTHY

An amazing machine

The human body is an amazing machine. The complexity of the body systems indicates an intelligent designer. One of the most amazing features is the way in which food, (our fuel), actually gets converted into energy, to keep the machine running. The human cell is extremely complex. It is the basic structural and functional unit of life. In the human body there are 100 trillion or so cells all with specialised functions. Within the cells are mitochondria, sometimes called 'powerplants', or the powerhouse of the cell. They are capable of converting energy in food to a form that cells can use.[1]

Such an amazingly complex machine deserves the best care and the best fuel. The Bible has a good deal to say about the fuel we should put into our bodies. It is advice from the One who created us.

Relevant today?

The Bible gives some sound advice on health. Many people would say that the dietary laws of the Old Testament were symbolic, and had no real connection with health. However, today there is much evidence to show that many of the dietary laws were actually set down by God for the physical health of His people, and not merely as ceremonial rituals.

"If you listen carefully to the voice of the Lord your God and do what is right in His eyes, if you pay attention to His commands and keep all His decrees, I will not bring on you any of these diseases…" (Exodus 15:26)

The Bible gives instructions for health that are now known to be scientifically and medically sound. For instance, lepers were instructed to live outside the city walls and not to come into contact with the general population. The fact that certain diseases were contagious was unknown to the world at the time, but we find instructions in the Bible to send away from the camp anyone who had a skin disease or discharge.

The Bible also warns against eating animal fat.
"It shall be a perpetual statute for your generations throughout all your dwellings, that you eat neither fat nor blood." (Leviticus 3:17)

These days we know that too much fat is not conducive to good health. The eating of blood is not recommended because unless meat is cooked extremely well, the viruses and disease-causing bacteria present in the flesh of the animal cannot be destroyed. That's bad news for people who enjoy their steak rare!

One Bible character who chose pure and wholesome food was Daniel. He chose to eat only vegetables and refused the rich food from the king's table. His three friends Shadrach, Meshach and Abednego did the same. After ten days of eating only vegetables and drinking water, they were stronger and healthier than all those who had been eating the royal food. From then on the guard let them continue to eat vegetables instead of eating what the king provided. (Daniel chapter 1)

Our responsibility

It is our personal responsibility to look after our body.
"Do you not know that your body is a temple of the Holy Spirit, who is in you, whom

you have received from God?" (1 Corinthians 6:19)

We all have responsibility to make wise choices and decisions. Not everything is good for us. Let's be positive about the delicious, wholesome food that God provided for us in the Garden of Eden!

"All things are lawful for me but not all things are expedient." (1 Corinthians 10:23)

Should we eat meat?

In the Garden of Eden, Adam and Eve and all the animals lived purely on a plant food diet. God says, "I give you every seed-bearing plant on the face of the whole earth, and every tree that has fruit with seed in it. They will be yours for food." (Genesis 1:29) This was God's perfect will.

However, after the great flood, permission was given to eat certain meats because there was no plant food around for a while. Meat became the emergency rations. We therefore can conclude that before the great flood, humanity was quite capable of living without meat entirely.

We can all benefit by eating a predominantly plant food diet. We are now living in an age in which there is a wide range of plant foods available to us, from every corner of the earth. Yet most people in Western society choose a diet that is predominantly animal products.

This kind of diet makes the body susceptible to degenerative diseases, including heart disease, cancer, diabetes, arthritis and osteoporosis. Meat lacks the plant chemicals for fighting disease and building the immune system. Feeling fit and healthy is not the measuring stick for good health. Degenerative diseases can creep us on us as we age, without warning signs. Have you ever heard of a person who has been healthy all their life, then suddenly dies of a heart attack, or suddenly contracts cancer? This is all too common. Prevention must begin early in life, and become a way of life. This is the only way to be healthy in later years.

There are popular fad diet theories around that claim that because we are all different, some people of a particular metabolic type must eat meat for good health. The theory claims that we must go back to the diet of our ancestors and that if your ancestors ate meat, then you will supposedly do better on a meat-based diet. Simarlily it claims that if your ancestors ate plants, then you will do better on a plant-based diet. This popular theory is bad news for those who think their ancestors ate meat. The truth is, the original ancestors of the whole human race ate a purely plant-food diet. Yes, we can all do better by eating the diet of our ancestors – the 'Garden of Eden' diet.

How much meat is too much? We must remember that meat is a high-protein food. Eating meat every day places strain on the body's organs during the digestive process. For those who maintain meat in their diet, try eating plant foods only for 3 days a week, and on other days, eat only a small amount of meat once per day.

Escaping the rat-race

Stress is a major cause of illness. Stress may not be caused by a specific event, but may be a result of the cumulative impact of our environment upon our lives. Although most of us are aware of the importance of adequate rest, recreation, exercise and good diet, the busyness of life often crowds out the things of most importance. Being in the 'rat-race' has a major effect upon our bodies.

"We have less time for meals than we once did, and we do not always have them when we should. We cook the wrong foods, or the right foods in the wrong way, to save time. We fail to give ourselves time to properly digest what we have eaten. Meals are sandwiched between other activities. We fit in eating when there is a gap, or when our work schedule insists we stop to eat. Meals are all too often 'grabbed' or 'snatched'; drinks are 'downed' and food 'bolted'. We no longer 'partake' of meals but abruptly 'have' them, and there are always 'fast-food' stores to help us along. Artificial products and artificially preserved foods take over our cupboards and refrigerators. Harmful additives are mixed into natural foods to extend their supermarket 'shelf-life'. All this impairs our health and capacity to cope." [2]

In order to live life to its full potential, we need to discover the creative possibilities that lie in doing less, live at a more measured pace and act in a less regulated way. We must seek to escape the rat-race, recover our equilibrium and discover a different way of life.

How do we become more tranquil? The first step is to become quite clear about God's path for our life. Say with the Psalm writer, "My times are in Your hands". There is no doubt that as we seek His priorities for our use of time, then He will give us the time. *3*

Setting time aside for rest, recreation and worshipping God, will do wonders for our health and well-being. A complete change from the daily work routine once a week is a biblical principle:
"Six days shalt thou labour..." (Exodus 20:6)
As we seek first God and His kingdom, then time for the most important things in life will be added to us. (Matthew 6:33) *4*

Emotional healing

Apart from the sheer pace of life, stress can be brought on by life's problems... breakdown in relationships, financial hardship and loss of loved-ones, to name a few. These problems may severely impact our emotional well-being. Many of today's lifestyle diseases have their roots in a trauma or emotional upset. When the body is under stress through trauma, or on-going emotional problems caused by that trauma, the immune system is compromised. Building the immune system through nutrition is essential, but will not be enough on its own. Everyone who suffers from on-going emotional problems should seek help in the form of counseling and prayer. It is important to release those problems by giving them to God, and to make a conscious effort to put the past behind. Give every new day to God, and trust Him to be in control of all your circumstances.

"Forget the former things; do not dwell on the past.
See I am doing a new thing!
I am making a way in the desert and streams in the wasteland," says the Lord. (Isaiah 43:18-19)

Food that heals

Food is very much a part of God's healing plan for today…even better, the right food may prevent us from getting sick in the first place!

We were made to be healthy. In God's perfect creation there was no sickness. You might be thinking that sickness today is inescapable because we now live in an imperfect world. As imperfect as it may be, there are ways to reclaim some of that original plan for perfect health. God wants us to be healthy. Obviously there could be nobody more worthy than our God, in whom to put our trust. But do we really believe it? Is He trustworthy in all things? Are we prepared to trust Him to heal us using the plants and herbs He created? We know His divine healing (supernatural healing), is available to us along with the amazing advances made in modern medicine. Why not natural healing too?

"Trust in the Lord with all your heart and lean not on your own understanding; in all your ways acknowledge Him and He will make your path straight." Proverbs 3:5-6

Unfortunately, very few people trust natural medicine at all, or even consider it useful in conjunction with what orthodox medicine has to offer. Many surrender all authority to orthodox medicine without giving natural healing a chance. They think that following a natural remedy is a little naive, based upon superstition and old wives' tales. They think of orthodox medicine, on the other hand, as being scientifically based. While many wonderful scientific discoveries have been made in the field of orthodox medicine, more and more discoveries are being made in the field of natural medicine, proving it to be scientifically sound.

Orthodox medicine treats the symptoms, often by means of a dose of antibiotics or removal of an ailing part. Natural medicine on the other hand tackles the underlying cause. Given time, and the right healing agents, the body has the ability to heal itself. Natural therapy can also provide preventative measures through the building up of the immune system. Taking supplements, (even when we are not sick), and consistently maintaining a healthy diet, will help our bodies fight off disease. Most orthodox medicine works by finding a remedy for the existing disease, rather than avoiding it.

There will be times when we need orthodox medicine (especially at times of emergency and for diagnosis), and times when natural medicine is the thing we need for a permanent cure. There are also times when both can be used together.

Train up a child

"Train up a child in the way he should go: and when he is old he will not depart from it." (Proverbs 22:6)

The home is the best place for teaching children the values of good health. By setting the example and carefully explaining the reasons for eating the right foods, children will be more cooperative about eating healthy food.

Abstaining from junk food will not really be a problem if you don't have it in the house. When children encounter junk food outside of the home situation, it won't be too much of a problem if you educate them on the dangers of eating it. (Also, make sure you feed them well before they go to birthday parties). Make sure they have a variety of delicious healthy food available in the home, and send food along to any social gatherings they attend.

Children love to be involved in the preparation of food. Although having the assistance of little hands is often more of a hindrance than help, learning to prepare food is an important part of the training process. The home is the perfect place for cooking lessons.

Parents have a responsibility to protect their children from the poisons that permeate much of our modern food. Just because certain foods are passed as 'safe' by a food protection authority does not mean that they actually are. They may not poison you in the short-term but will probably have long-term effects. Healthy food can build strong immunity against the number of rapidly increasing virus strains prevalent today. Who knows how severe these viruses will become in the future. One of the best things you can do for your children is to wean them off refined table sugar, fast food and junk food, and to ensure that they eat plenty of fresh fruit and vegetables.

One in every ten Australian children is obese and in need of medical attention, new data reveals. It also shows that 25% are in danger of becoming overweight. The causes are the eating of take-away food and junk food, not exercising, and too much T.V. Families are also too busy and there's less time to do active things together. Let's give our children good values...not just in moral terms, but in healthy living as well!

All things in moderation?

While this is generally a good motto, we should beware of applying it to things that are toxic. Most wouldn't agree that smoking is good in moderation. When it comes to things that are toxic, abstinence is the better way to go.

When someone has an ailment caused through diet, the best way to deal with the problem is to abstain from the food contributing to the ailment. For instance, people with allergies or colds should abstain from dairy products. People with heart disease should abstain from the bad fats. Yet how many times do we hear, "I hardly ever eat such and such", or "I eat very little of whatever." Moderation is not going to allow the body to heal itself. In these cases abstinence is the key.

The difficulty with eating junk food in moderation is that there is no measuring stick. How much is too much? Is it once a day or once a week? We can make our own standard to appease our conscience. 'Hardly ever' for some people might be once a week. For some it might be once a day. Rather than saying "all things in moderation", it is better to say, "some things in moderation and some things never."

Children are very susceptible to the effects of toxins. Toxins are responsible for ailments such as asthma, eczema and A.D.D. Read food labels. Buy a chart that decodes food additive numbers. Become aware of the toxins in processed food. The same applies to the toxins we put on our skin in terms of personal care products. Believe it or not, the toxins do get absorbed.

Invincible youth

Young people enjoy a high level of health and well-being simply because of their age. The 'invincibility of youth' is like a healthy bank account from which it is possible to make too many rash withdrawals. For such a person, the 'health account' eventually dries up, moving into debit. Reserves of vitality, energy and immunity become depleted with age, resulting in illness. Self-abuse comes at a cost.

All too often we eat and drink whatever tastes good, using the taste buds as the sole arbiter for what we allow into our stomachs! Let's not wait until we are older to get the wake-up call. May be it will be too late. We don't have to die of a degenerative disease. How much better it is to live a long and healthy life, and die simply because our time has run out! (Job 5:26)

Endnotes

1. Wardlaw, Hampl & Di Silvestro, *Perspectives in Nutrition*, 6th edition, USA, 2004, p. 34
2. Banks, Robert, *The Tyranny of Time*, Aust., 1939, pp. 40-41
3. Ibid. p. 210
4. Ibid

part B:
RECIPES

CONTENTS

INTRODUCTION..121

1. Health Products and Ingredients........................124

2. Useful Equipment for your Kitchen......................128

3. Butter and Cream Substitutes...........................130
    - 130 Savoury cashew spread
    - 131 Spicy cashew spread
    - 131 Almond cream
    - 131 Avocado
    - 131 Carob and date spread
    - 132 Date butter
    - 132 Houmus
    - 132 Nut cream
    - 133 Rice cream

4. Salad Dressings & Dips...133
    - 133 Oil and lemon dressing
    - 133 Mayonnaise
    - 133 Sunflower dressing
    - 134 Avocado dressing
    - 134 Red kidney bean dip
    - 134 Guacamole dip
    - 135 Eggplant and tahini dip
    - 135 Savoury cashew dip

5. Milk Substitutes..135
    - 135 Nut Milk
    - 136 Rice milk fruit smoothiie

6. Breakfast Foods..136
    - 136 S.L.A.P.
    - 136 Fruit salad

7. **Snacks**..136
   - 136   Toasted Sandwiches
   - 137   Buckwheat Waffles
   - 137   Oatmeal waffles
   - 137   Rice-Oat Waffles
   - 138   French Toast
   - 138   Potato Savouries
   - 138   Tomato and Chive Twists
   - 139   Granola
   - 139   Toasted Muesli
   - 139   Sesame Crunch

8. **Soups**..140
   - 140   Pea Soup
   - 140   Minestrone
   - 141   Red lentil and potato soup
   - 141   Bean and Whole Grain Soup
   - 142   Pumpkin Soup
   - 142   Potato Soup
   - 142   Potato and corn soup
   - 143   Clear Vegetable Soup with Tempeh

9. **Vegetarian Main Meals**...143
   Salads:..143
   - 143   Chunky Salad
   - 144   Chick Pea Salad
   - 144   Tabouleh Salad
   - 145   Rice Salad
   - 145   Rice and avocado salad
   - 146   Potato Salad
   - 146   Avocado Salad
   - 146   Coleslaw
   - 147   Mung bean salad
   - 147   Spinach avocado salad
   - 147   Bean salad
   - 148   Lentil salad
   - 148   Beetroot salad

Vegetables: 148
148   Home-made Tomato and Vegetable Puree
149   Ratatouille
149   Curried vegetables and brown rice
150   Nut stir-fry
150   Baked Potato Chips
151   Chinese Stir-fry
151   Thai style stir-fry
152   Tomato and Beans with Greens
152   Cauliflower in White Sauce
153   Sweet Potato au Gratin

Stews, Casseroles and Hot Pots 153
153   Moussaka
154   Eggplant Italian
154   Mexican Chili Beans
155   Mexican Tortilla
155   Bean and Vegetable Hot Pot
156   Pumpkin Hot Pot
156   Haricot Beans in Tomato Sauce
156   Bean Stew
156   Spiced Chick Peas
157   Red Lentil Dahl
158   Split pea dahl
158   Layered Vegetable Casserole

Pasta and Pizza: 159
159   Lentil Bolognaise
159   Lentil Lasagne
160   Vegetable Lasagne
160   Pesto with Pasta
161   Creamy Pasta
161   Vegetable Pasta Sauce
162   Mushroom Pasta Sauce
162   Pizza

Burgers, Pancakes and Vegie-loaves: 163
- 163 Vegie Burgers
- 163 Curried vegie-burgers
- 164 Lentil Burgers
- 164 Quinoa Burgers
- 165 Tempeh Balls
- 165 Falafel
- 166 Spinach pancakes
- 166 Corn Fritters
- 166 Potato and Corn Patties
- 167 Tempeh Vege Loaf
- 167 Nut Burgers
- 168 Oatmeal-almond loaf

Grains: 168
- 168 Quinoa Stuffed Capsicum
- 169 Millet Bake
- 169 Barley and Zucchini Bake
- 170 Buckwheat and mushrooms

Pies and Pastries: 170
- 170 Nut Pastry
- 171 Potato Pastry
- 171 Shepherd's Pie
- 171 Lentil Pie
- 172 Mushroom and Lentil Pie
- 172 Arame Rolls
- 173 Spring Rolls
- 173 Pumpkin Pasties
- 174 Spinach and Rice Pie
- 174 Winter Pie

Egg Dishes: 175
- 175 Zucchini Slice
- 175 Quiche
- 175 Speedy Omelette

10. Fish..........176
- 176 Baked Fish and Corn Casserole
- 176 Baked Fish and Potato Casserole
- 177 Fish Soup
- 177 Fish Pasta Sauce
- 178 Fish Cakes
- 178 Salmon with Rice and Stir-fried Vegetables
- 178 Fish, Potato and Rice Casserole

11. Fast Foods..........179
- 179 Rice
- 179 Quick Stir-Fry
- 180 Beans
- 180 Frozen Food
- 180 Toasted Sandwiches
- 180 Pizza

12. Sweet Treats for Special Occasions..........180

Slices:..........180
- 180 Muesli Slice
- 181 Oatmeal Slice
- 181 Gluten-free slice
- 182 Carrot Slice

Cookies and Truffles:..........182
- 182 Carob Cookies
- 183 Banana Date Cookies
- 183 Apple & date Cookies
- 184 Gingerbread cookies
- 184 Truffles
- 184 Fruit Balls

Desserts and afternoon teas:..........185
- 185 Nut Pastry
- 185 Custard
- 186 Fruit Pies
- 186 Lemon Pie
- 186 Pumpkin Pie

187 Frozen Fruit Sorbet
187 Carrot Cake
187 Apple and Raisin Cake
188 Hot Fruit Salad
188 Sago Delight
188 Apricot Delight
189 Fruit Jelly
189 Fruit Crumble
190 Creamed Rice with Dates

Cakes:..190
190 Porridge Cake
190 Apple Cake
191 Fruit Cake
191 Eggless Fruit Cake
192 Coconut Fruit Cake
192 Sultana Muffins
192 Apple Muffins
193 Dried Fruit Muffins
193 Fresh Fruit Muffins
193 Carob Muffins

13. Bread..194
194 Wholemeal Bread

14. Thermomix Recipes..194
195 Coleslaw
195 Beetroot salad
195 Minestrone
196 Chick pea soup
196 Thick red lentils
196 Savoury cashew spread
197 Nut burgers
197 Custard
198 Agar fruit jelly
198 Taiwanese porridge

INTRODUCTION

These recipes have been designed to maintain and promote health. Many of the recipes in this book have been instrumental in my husband's recovery from lymphoma, a cancer of the lymph system. The recipes eliminate potentially harmful ingredients, are designed for maximum nutritional benefits and at the same time provide delicious taste experiences! Recipes have been created or modified to stay within the guidelines of a recovery diet. Suffering from a life-threatening disease however, is not a prerequisite for following the eating plan suggested in this book. We have found it beneficial for the whole family, and look upon it as a way for healthy people to stay healthy. Prevention is better than cure!

Main course recipes should be served with plenty of fresh vegetables, either raw or lightly steamed. For those with cancer, remember 80% raw plant food at every meal. That is, fruit for breakfast and salad for lunch and dinner. For the other 20%, concentrate on ingredients that provide a good protein source, such as the nuts, seeds and legumes. Select recipes accordingly. Do not snack in between meals, but rather, make your own juices.

For those with cancer, Max Gerson suggests that no animal protein be eaten for the first four months. Thereafter, add a small amount of pure organic animal products.

For those without cancer, but want to avoid it, there are many food ideas in this book that will cater for the whole family, and provide substitutes for the things you would be better off cutting out. Remember that everyone benefits by a diet that majors on raw plant foods.

Always keep a good balance between proteins, fats and carbohydrates, whether you are sick or healthy. For lunch and dinner, complement your raw salad with something from each of these categories:

Protein: lentils, dried beans, chick peas, nuts, seeds, free-range eggs, organic natural yoghurt, sardines or wild salmon

Carbohydrate: lentils, dried beans, chick peas, brown rice, potatoes, sweet potatoes, millet, buckwheat, quinoa, oats

Fat: avocado, cold-pressed olive oil, coconut oil, nuts and seeds, free-range eggs, 'safe' fish

The past decade has given rise to similar popular recipe books, based on the principle that our food should be our medicine. Many people are being awakened to the need to 'eat our way to health'. However this book attempts to go one step further than previous health recipe books. It is more particular in the use of ingredients, aiming to eliminate the ingredients that have a potentially harmful impact upon our health. It provides tasty substitutes for all ingredients eliminated, making the food so delicious, while at the same time extremely healthy. Whenever I share these dishes with conventional eaters at social functions, I am constantly asked for the recipes!

TOP 10 RECIPES

Most people know how to prepare raw salads, so you don't really need recipes for these. However you may find the cooked section of the meal more challenging. The following ten recipes are my family favourites, and a good place to start.

1. Savoury Cashew Spread (very versatile!)
2. Lentil Bolognaise
3. Lentil Lasagne
4. Spiced Chick Peas

5. Mexican Beans
6. Split Pea Soup
7. Nut Burgers
8. Quiche
9. Zucchini Slice
10. Muesli Slice

Recipes in this book contain:
- NO sugar
- NO heated oil except for cold-pressed olive oil and coconut oil
- NO refined table salt
- NO preservatives or artificial colourings and flavourings
- NO red meat or chicken
- NO dairy products except for organic natural yoghurt

WEIGHTS AND MEASURES
Weights are in grams.

30 g.	=	1 ounce
125 g.	=	4 ounces
250 g.	=	8 ounces
375 g.	=	12 ounces
500 g.	=	1 pound

Liquid measures are in mls.

30 ml.	=	1 fl. ounces
125 ml.	=	4 fl. ounces
250 ml.	=	8 fl. ounces or ½ pint, or a standard cup measure.
500 ml.	=	1 pint

Oven Temperatures
150 degrees C = 250 degrees F = gas mark 2 (slow)
180 degrees C = 350 degrees F = gas mark 4 (moderate)
200 degrees C = 400 degrees F = gas mark 6 (moderately hot)

A word about soy
The use of soy products has become controversial. There is some concern that processed, unfermented soy products can cause hormone imbalance, depress thyroid function and block mineral absorption. Soy milk has therefore not

been used in these recipes. Fermented soy products like tempeh, miso and tamari however are safe. Rice milk may be used as an alternative to soy milk, if the rice milk does not contain canola oil.

A word about wheat

Many people have wheat allergies, and most of us would be better off choosing other grains. Please choose from the wide variety of flour available in health shops and supermarkets. Brown rice flour, buckwheat flour and millet flour are all good alternatives. Pasta does not have to be wheat pasta. Rice pasta and corn pasta are both available in health shops or health sections of your supermarket.

1. HEALTH PRODUCTS AND INGREDIENTS

These products are available from health shops and health sections of your supermarket:

1. Celtic salt

This is an unrefined, non-toxic, natural salt, which is hand harvested from the sea. It is grey in appearance and not white. It is granulated, and dissolves in liquid foods. For seasoning food at the table, a grinder is necessary.

2. Herbamare herbal salt (Bioforce/Vogel)

This may be sprinkled directly on to food.

3. Plantaforce vegetable stock (Bioforce/Vogel)

This is available in both cube form and paste form. Made from pure vegetable stock and does not contain refined salt or MSG.

4. Miso

Miso is a savoury paste made from fermented soya beans. It may be added to soups or stir-fried vegetables. It can also be used as a spread.

5. Hungarian sweet paprika

This is a pepper or chili alternative. It is made from capsicum and does not aggravate the lining of the stomach.

6. Tempeh
Tempeh is another fermented soya bean product which can be used in stir fries or in casserole dishes. Unlike tofu, tempeh has a more savoury taste. It is a good source of protein.

7. Kelpamare kelp sauce (Bioforce/Vogel)
This is a delicious, healthy sauce containing seaweed, and tastes similar to soy sauce.

8. Tamari
This is a healthier form of soy sauce, lower in salt.

9. Arame
This is a form of dried Japanese seaweed. It needs to be soaked and boiled for 15 minutes.

10. Brown rice flour
This thickener, a good substitute for custard powder or refined cornflour.

11. Cornflour or maize flour
Check that the brand of cornflour you buy is made from corn and not wheat.

12. Burghul
This grain is delicious in salads.

13. Quinoa
Pronounced "keen-wah"
This is a whole grain from South America. It contains more quality protein than any other grain, and provides an essential amino acid balance. It is light and easy to digest, and quick and easy to prepare.

14. Fruit juice concentrate
This is a thick syrup which can be used in place of cane sugar. Apple juice or pear juice are most suitable.

15. Agar agar
This is a seaweed extract which can be used as a stabilising agent in jellies and ice-cream and other cold desserts.

16. Tahini
Tahini is a paste made from sesame seeds, high in calcium. It can be used as a spread, or in cooking, as a replacement for refined oil.

17. 'Good' bread
Bread without 471 or 472, (animal fat). Also low in salt and free from preservatives and sugar. Try and find bread that doesn't contain wheat. Organic, sour rye dough bread is preferable. 'Country Life', an Australian company, make a good organic sour-rye dough bread.

18. 'Good' flour
Shouldn't be too refined and shouldn't contain bleach. Should be low in salt. Organic is preferable. Organic spelt flour is quite good. This is made from an ancient variety of wheat that contains vitamin B17. It is not necessary to use wheat flour. Millet flour and buckwheat flour, both containing vitamin B17, are two good alternatives.

19. Dried fruit
Dried fruit without preservative 220 can be found in health shops.

GUIDELINES FOR COOKING DRIED BEANS, CHICK PEAS AND LENTILS
Soak dried beans, chick peas and lentils overnight. For lentils, soak in boiling water for 10 minutes as an alternative to soaking in cold water overnight. After soaking, rinse all beans and lentils thoroughly. The reason for soaking and rinsing is not only to reduce cooking time, but also to remove the outer substance, which can cause wind in the digestive system.

Cooking beans, chick peas and lentils in a saucepan will take less time than in a crock-pot. A crock-pot, however, has the advantage of unattended cooking. It does not boil over and food does not stick to the bottom. A crock-pot is therefore more convenient if you have the time. If using a saucepan, a heat-reducing mesh ring is excellent to help stop boiling over. If using a crock-pot, you need to cover your ingredients with 2/3 water. i.e. Fill the pot with 1/3 soaked legumes to 2/3 water.

Soaking and cooking times for beans chick peas and lentils:
Times are for boiling on stove. Crock-pot takes at least double time.

Black-eye beans; haricot/navy beans; red kidney beans, chick peas:
Soak 3 hours, or over night. Cook for 2 hours.
Lentils (brown or green): Soak 10 minutes, (boiling water), or overnight in cold water. Rinse and drain. Add fresh water. Cook 1 hour.
Lentils (red): Soak 5 minutes, (boiling water). Cook 30 minutes.

Cooking time for brown rice:
Brown rice needs to be boiled for 35 minutes. A cooking mat, sold for the purpose of placing on the hot plate, will stop the rice sticking to the bottom of the saucepan. Cooked brown rice can be stored in a glass jar in the fridge for 2-3 days and heated with Tamari or Kelp Sauce as required.

HERBS, SPICES AND SEASONINGS
Some people prefer highly flavoured foods. Others prefer their food less spicy or salty. Eating in a healthy way does not mean that all seasoning has to be eliminated. I have eliminated certain spices such as black pepper, and chosen seasonings that do not aggravate the stomach. If the recipes in this book are not tasty enough for you, simply add more than the suggested amount.

Celtic salt - A healthy substitute for refined salt.

Stock cubes – Should be all vegetable and contain no MSG.

Onions and garlic - As well as providing excellent flavour, onions and garlic are antioxidants. Garlic in particular is a natural antibiotic.

Herbs and spices - Herbs are better fresh than dried. If you don't have space in the garden, try growing them inside in pots. You will need to replace them more often, but plants are not too expensive. Although there are many herbs available, these are the ones that I use the most:

Sweet paprika is a good substitute for pepper. Choose the Hungarian variety, which is made from capsicum and not from chilies.

Basil, oregano and ***thyme*** are excellent herbs for Italian flavouring.

Dill goes very nicely with fish.

Parsley is high in iron and suitable in many dishes.

Mint adds subtle flavour to chick pea salads or grain salads.

Cumin, turmeric and ***coriander*** give excellent flavour in Indian style dishes.

Bay leaves give excellent flavour to bean or vegetables stews and hot pots.

Lemon balm or ***lemon grass*** gives lemon flavour to spreads and salads.

Chives are great for a mild onion flavour in a fresh salad.

Rosemary, sage and ***thyme*** go nicely together in vegetable and lentil burgers.

Cinnamon, cloves, ginger and ***nutmeg*** are delicious in desserts, slices and cakes.

Root ginger is excellent in Chinese style dishes.

Nutmeg can also be used to enhance the flavour of savoury foods such as pumpkin or mushrooms.

2. USEFUL EQUIPMENT FOR YOUR KITCHEN

1. Food processor
This has a large blade that chops food very finely. It is useful for making sauces, nut spreads, slices, quiches, pureed soup and pastry. For a very fine blend you need to process the food with liquid.

2. Blender
This is useful for making purees. It blends food more finely than a food processor. You need a blender with a strong motor for blending nuts with liquid.

3. Coffee grinder
A small electric coffee grinder grinds nuts and seeds very well. Ground nuts and seeds can be sprinkled on breakfast cereals or desserts. The coffee grinder will also grind nuts and sunflower seeds for slices. Alternatively, hand grinders are available from some kitchen shops.

4. Thermomix multi-function food processor
This machine takes the place of a food processor, blender, coffee grinder and many other appliances. It will chop, mix, pulverise, grind, grate, puree, cook, steam and weigh. Made from stainless steel, it is extremely durable and will grind nuts, seeds and even grains. It prepares soups, stews and stir-fry dishes from raw ingredients, while you get on with doing something else. Thermomix recipes have been included at the back of this book. (Available from www.thermomix.com.au)

5. Small bench-top oven
This is useful for heating that odd slice of left-over pie without using a microwave. (Preparing food in microwaves destroys food value and adds to the risk of cancer.) You can also cook casseroles, chips, baked potatoes and other vegetables in a small oven, avoiding the expense of heating your large oven. A small oven heats up quickly and is therefore more efficient.

6. Crock-pot
This is excellent for soups, lentils and pulses. Food cooks slowly, taking at least double the time of a saucepan on the stove, but the advantage is that you can set it going in the morning making sure your water level is high enough, ($1/3$ food to $2/3$ liquid), and you can forget about it for 6 to 8 hours. Food won't boil over and the contents won't boil dry. Neither will the contents stick to the bottom of the pot!

7. Pyrex baking dishes
These are clear oven-proof glass dishes, essential for making slices and should be used in place of slab tins. Because recipes use no butter or margarine, mixture baked in slab tins will not hold together properly and will crack. The pyrex baking dishes do not need greasing and can be cleaned easily if left to soak several hours before washing. Slab tins are also prone to rust whereas pyrex is not.

8. Juicer

High quality centrifuge juicers or press juicers are best. These are usually available through health shops and not department stores. Such juicers extract more juice, leave dryer pulp and maintain the oxygen level in the juice for longer.

3. BUTTER, CREAM AND CHEESE SUBSTITUTES

Nuts are used in many recipes as substitutes for butter and cream. Nuts contain high levels of natural oils so make an excellent substitute when used in moderation. For people with allergic reactions to nuts, sunflower seeds can be used instead. For best nutritional value, nuts should be raw, and not the roasted, salted variety.

All dishes containing ground nuts should be kept in the refrigerator for a maximum of 3 days. After this time, oil from the nuts can become rancid. Rancid oils cause cancer. Nut spreads can be frozen in small quantities.

Nut spreads can be made in either a food processor or a strong blender. A blender gives a smoother spread. If using a blender, start with liquid and gradually add nuts.

Savoury Cashew Spread

1½ cups cashews (200 g.)
1 cup water
3 heaped teasp. arrowroot or cornflour
1 teasp. Celtic salt
¼ teasp. sweet paprika
1 teasp. onion powder

1. Place nuts in food processor and blend until fine.
2. Place cold water in saucepan on stove. Add arrowroot and whisk while it is coming to the boil. This makes a thick, smooth paste.
3. Blend the arrowroot paste with the ground nuts in the food processor. Blend well.

If using a blender, start with the arrowroot paste and add nuts gradually to paste while blending. *Note: Torula yeast is non-living and is not the kind of yeast that can cause candida*

Spicy Cashew Spread
1 cup water
3 heaped teasp. arrowroot or cornflour
1½ cups cashews (200 g.)
1 teasp. Celtic salt
2 tablesp. grated onion
piece capsicum
¼ clove garlic
1 dessertsp. lemon juice (or ½ teasp. lemon grass herb)
1 teasp. sweet paprika

1. Place nuts in food processor and blend until fine.
2. Place cold water in saucepan. Add arrowroot and whisk as the mixture thickens and comes to the boil. Cool slightly.
3. Add the thickened arrowroot mixture to nuts in food processor. Add all other ingredients and blend well.

This recipe makes a fairly thick paste suitable for spreading. If you require a thinner paste for pouring, use more water. If using a blender, start with liquid and add nuts gradually while blending.

Almond Cream
1 cup almonds
½ cup dates
1½ cups water

1. Place ingredients in blender and cover with water.
2. Blend until smooth.

Use to pour over fruit, or mixture of chopped nuts and seeds.

Avocado
This is an excellent substitute for butter. Spread your salad sandwich thickly with ripe avocado and you will not miss the butter!

Carob and Date Spread
8 dates (softened in a little water on stove)
¾ cup tahini
1 tablesp. carob powder
¼ cup orange juice

1. Place all ingredients in blender.
2. Blend. Add extra liquid if mixture is too stiff.
This is a substitute for chocolate spread.

Date Butter
½ cup water or rice milk
½ cup dates
¼ cup almonds
few drops of natural vanilla

1. Heat dates in water on stove until soft.
2. Blend all ingredients in blender. Add a few extra drops of water if too stiff.
Spread on bread or waffles. Also use as cake frosting. For carob flavour, dissolve carob powder in boiling water and add.

Houmus
2 cups chick peas, soaked, rinsed and cooked for 1 hour.
juice of ½ lemon
1 teasp. Celtic salt
3 leaves fresh basil
fresh parsley/chives
2 tablesp. tahini
1 cup water

1. Place all in blender.
2. Blend. Add a little extra water if needed to make a smooth paste. Blend again.
This spread may be refrigerated 3-4 days, or frozen.

Nut Cream
½ cup nuts (e.g. almonds, cashews or hazelnuts)
1 cup water

1. Place water in a blender.
2. Gradually add nuts while blending.
Use to pour on bread, toast, pancakes or waffles. Delicious with honey or stewed fruit.

Rice Cream

1½ cups cooked rice
½ cup raw cashews
2 tablesp. honey
1 cup water

1. Place all ingredients in blender.
2. Blend.
Served with fruit or mixture of chopped nuts and seeds.

4. SALAD DRESSINGS AND DIPS

Oil and Lemon Dressing

½ cup olive oil
1 teasp. honey
1 dessertsp. lemon juice
Mix together or shake.

Mayonnaise

½ cup water
1 level tablesp. brown rice flour
1 egg
1 teasp. turmeric powder
½ teasp. sweet paprika
1 teasp. onion powder
1 dessertsp. olive oil
½ teasp. Celtic salt
1 teasp. grated lemon rind
1 tablesp. lemon juice
1 teasp. honey

1. Whisk rice flour, egg and water in saucepan over heat, and bring to the boil. Cool.
2. Place this thickened mixture into a blender with all ingredients and blend.

Sunflower Dressing

½ cup sunflower seeds
1 tablesp. lemon juice

¾ cup water
1 teasp. onion powder
1 teasp. Celtic salt

Blend until smooth.
This can be used as a substitute for cream on baked potatoes.

Avocado Dressing
1 ripe avocado, peeled and core removed
½ cup water
1 tablesp. lemon juice
1 clove garlic or ½ salad onion
1 teasp. Celtic salt

Blend until smooth.

Red Kidney Bean Dip
2 cups red kidney beans, cooked and drained
1 cup tomatoes
1 onion, chopped
1 tablesp. tomato paste
½ teasp. sweet paprika
1 teasp. onion powder
1 teasp. Celtic salt

1. Cook the tomatoes and onions with salt for 10 minutes in a saucepan.
2. Blend all ingredients in a food processor.
3. Warm through in a saucepan on the stove.

Guacamole Dip
2 ripe avocados
1 tablesp. lemon juice
1 clove garlic, crushed
1 spring onion
1 large tomato, skinned and chopped
¼ teasp. sweet paprika
2 tablesp. fresh coriander, chopped
¼ teasp. Celtic salt

1. Cut the avocados in half and remove stones.
2. Blend avocado flesh in food processor with all other ingredients.
To make without a food processor, mash with a fork.
Serve as a dip or spread on pita bread.

Eggplant and Tahini Dip

2 large eggplants
1 clove garlic, crushed
2 tablesp. tahini
1 tablesp. lemon juice
½ teasp. Celtic salt
½ teasp. sweet paprika

1. Prick eggplants and steam, or bake in casserole dish in oven, with lid on.
2. Cut eggplant into slices and remove skin.
3. Blend eggplant in food processor with all other ingredients.
Serve warm on pita bread or with rice crackers.

Savoury Cashew Dip

Follow the recipe for 'Savoury Cashew Spread', or 'Spicy Cashew Spread' *(Butter, Cream and Cheese Substitutes section)*.
Serve as a dip.

5. MILK SUBSTITUTES

Western society has become dependent on milk as a staple food. However, we still have the highest statistics on osteoporosis. We do not need milk. Once you have exchanged the traditional milk and cereal breakfast for the raw fruit/nut/seed breakfast, and eliminated traditional tea and coffee, you will not find the need to consume milk. However nut/rice milk fruit smoothies make a good snack, especially for children. Rice, nut milk or fresh fruit juice can also be used on home-made muesli, and eaten any time of day.

Nut Milk

½ cup raw cashews or almonds
2 cups water.
Place in blender with a little water, then add more water.

Rice Milk Fruit Smoothie
1 tablesp. cooked rice
¼ cup raw cashews
1 teasp.. honey
1 teasp. coconut oil
1 cup water

1. Place all ingredients in blender.
2. Blend.
3. Add banana, mango or berries. Blend again.
If using commercial rice milk, use one without canola oil.

6. BREAKFAST FOODS

S.L.A.P.
1 dessertsp. each of the following:
sunflower seeds
linseeds (flax seeds)
almonds (roughly chopped firstly by hand)
pepitas (pumpkin seed kernels)

Grind in an electric coffee grinder. Place in a bowl with a little grape juice and coconut oil. Stir well. Add chopped fresh juicy fruits.

Fruit Salad
Start the day with a bowl of fresh fruit. This is an excellent habit to develop in children. Use any juicy fruits, but not bananas or melons at this time of day. Paw paw and pineapple contain important enzymes, so should be included. Fruit in the morning helps the elimination process. Raw nuts and seeds can be eaten with the fruit, and provide sustenance.

7. SNACKS
These snacks make good week-end lunch ideas for children.

Toasted Sandwiches
Use a regular sandwich maker or jaffle maker.
1. Spread outside of the bread with Savoury Cashew Spread . (See Butter, Cream and Cheese Substitutes).

2. Spread the cashew spread inside the sandwiches too, along with filling if desired.
Suggested fillings: avocado, tomato and celery; cooked lentils or beans in tomato sauce;

The cashew spread does not stick to the sandwich maker and replaces the need for butter or margarine.

Buckwheat Waffles
½ cup unbleached plain flour
½ cup buckwheat flour
1 cup rice milk or water

1. Whisk ingredients together.
2. Pour into waffle maker and cook for 3 minutes.

This makes enough for 3 waffles; (12 quarter segments). Serve as sweet or savoury.
Suggested toppings: stewed apple; honey; fruit sorbet or nut cream; Mexican chilli beans. May be used for pancake mixture.

Oatmeal Waffles
1¾ cups water
1 tablesp. fruit juice concentrate
1½ cups rolled oats
½ teasp. Celtic salt

1. Blend.
2. Pour into waffle maker and cook 3 minutes.

Rice-Oat Waffles
3 cups water
2 tablesp. fruit juice concentrate
½ cup cashews
1 cup rolled oats
1¼ cup barley flour
1 teasp. vanilla
1 cup cooked brown rice
¼ cup cornmeal or cornflour

½ teasp. Celtic salt

Blend and cook in waffle maker 3 minutes.

French Toast
1 cup chick peas, soaked and rinsed
1½ cups water
¼ cup cashews
½ teasp. Celtic salt
herbs

1. Place all ingredients in blender or food processor and blend.
2. Dip bread in blended mixture.
3. Fry in electric frypan without oil, or cook in sandwich maker. Add tomato topping.

Potato Savouries
1 cup flour
1 cup mashed potato
½ cup water to mix

1. Mix dry ingredients and potato together and add enough water to make a dough.
2. Roll out as pastry, but thicker, (about ½ cm.)
3. Use a round cookie cutter to cut out shapes.
4. Place rounds on to an oven tray and top with avocado, tomato, savoury cashew spread or any favourite toppings.
5. Bake in a moderate oven for 10-12 minutes.

Tomato and Chive Twists
Use the above 'potato pastry' but cut into strips instead of rounds. Mix some tomato and onion puree, tomato paste and chives. Add other herbs if desired. Spread the mixture over the strips and twist. Place on baking tray in twisted lengths and bake as above.

Granola
Place in a mixing bowl:
½ cup sunflower seeds

4 cups oats
½ cup sesame seeds
¼ cup chopped nuts
Place in blender and blend:
1 large banana
few drops of natural vanilla essence
8 dates, softened in a little boiling water

1. Add blended ingredients to dry ingredients.
2. Spread on to an oven tray. Bake 140 degrees for 2 hours. Check and stir now and again.
3. Serve with nut cream or rice cream from 'Butter, Cream and Cheese Substitutes'. Alternatively serve with rice milk, organic natural yoghurt or fruit juice. This recipe, and the following, make a good afternoon or lunch snack for children.

Toasted Muesli
3 cups oats
½ cup oat bran
1 cup flaked almonds
½ cup sunflower seeds
½ cup sesame seeds
½ cup dried fruit

1. Spread oats, oat bran and almonds over surface of an oven tray or large oven proof dish.
2. Bake 30 minutes at 150 degrees, stirring occasionally.
3. When cool, place in mixing bowl. Add all other ingredients.
4. Serve with nut cream or rice cream from section 3 or with rice milk, natural yoghurt or fruit juice.

Sesame Crunch
1 cup rolled oats
½ cup sesame seeds
½ cup coconut or oat bran
1 teasp. olive oil or coconut oil
1 tablesp. honey

1. Mix all ingredients together in a large saucepan and stir for a minute over a low heat, just until oil and honey have blended through.
2. Spread out mixture in a shallow oven-proof baking dish.
3. Bake in moderate oven for 10 minutes. Remove from oven and stir, then bake a further 5 minutes.
4. Spoon mixture into a glass jar for storage. Eat from a snack cup with a spoon. No need to add milk or any liquid.

8. SOUPS

Pea Soup
2 cups dried split peas, rinsed and soaked
1 large onion
1 carrot
1 potato
1 stick of celery
2 teasp. Celtic salt

1. Place peas in saucepan or crock-pot. Add water. Cover to twice depth of peas.
2. Simmer.
3. When peas are soft, add other vegetables and Celtic salt. Simmer for a further half an hour.

Minestrone
½ cup red kidney beans
½ cup black eye beans
1 grated onion
chopped vegetables as desired
1 teasp. dried Italian herbs or fresh basil and oregano
1 cup tomato puree
2 tablesp. tomato paste
1 teasp. Celtic salt

1. Rinse and soak beans.
2. Simmer beans in crock-pot until soft. Water level should be two-thirds above the beans.
3. Add all other ingredients. Add extra water if needed. Simmer until vegeta-

bles are cooked.
4. Add cooked pasta if desired.
You may prefer to cook tomato and vegetable mixture separately in a saucepan, and combine with beans cooked in crock-pot.

Red Lentil and Potato Soup
2 cups red lentils
1½ litres water
1 onion
1 piece capsicum
1 stick celery
2 diced potatoes
1 tablesp. tomato paste
2 teasp. Celtic salt

1. Soak, drain and rinse lentils.
2. Cook lentils and potato in 1 litre water until soft, (about 20 minutes)
3. Blend onion, capsicum and celery in ½ litre water and add to soup.
4. Add salt and tomato paste.
5. Cook for another 15 minutes.

Bean and Whole Grain Soup
2 cups mixed dried beans, rinsed and soaked
2 tablesp. each of the following:
buckwheat
millet
pearled barley
1 natural vegetable stock cube
1 teasp. Celtic salt
1 large onion, chopped or grated
2 cups chopped vegetables as desired

1. Place beans and wholegrains in crock-pot with adequate water.
2. Simmer about 6 hours.
3. Later, add onion, stock cube and salt.
4. Simmer until beans are soft. Add vegetables. Simmer a further hour.

Pumpkin Soup

900 g. raw pumpkin
1 medium potato
1 stick celery
1 onion
parsley
2 teasp. Celtic salt.
1 cup water

1. Steam all vegetables together.
2. Blend all vegetables together in food processor with Celtic salt and 1 cup water used for steaming.
3. Serve with chopped parsley.

Potato Soup

4 medium potatoes, steamed and mashed
1 onion
parsley
1 stick celery
1 small zucchini
1 teasp. Celtic salt
1 teasp. onion powder.
3 cups water

1. Blend onion, parsley, celery, zucchini, salt and onion powder in blender with 2 cups water.
2. Transfer to saucepan, bring to boil and simmer 5 minutes. Stir occasionally.
3. Add mashed potatoes and 1 cup water. Heat for another few minutes, while stirring.
4. Serve with extra chopped parsley.
Soup may be topped with a few slices of ripe avocado when serving. Steamed asparagus may also be added.

Potato and Corn Soup

2 corn cobs
3 medium potatoes or sweet potatoes
½ teasp. sweet paprika

1 onion
1 tablesp. olive oil
2 sticks celery
1 vegetable stock cube or 1 teasp. Celtic salt
1 tablesp. cornflour or brown rice flour
750 ml. Water

1. Dice potato, celery and remove husks from corn.
2. Place potato, celery and corn in large saucepan with water. Cook 10 minutes.
3. Remove corn cobs. Cool and strip corn. Put corn back in saucepan with potato and celery.
4. Chop onion and saute in olive oil. Add to saucepan.
5. Simmer a further 5 minutes, adding stock cube or Celtic salt, and sweet paprika.
Pasta may be added.

Clear Vegetable Soup with Tempeh
1 chopped onion
1 teasp. cold-pressed olive oil
3 cups chopped vegetables – various
60 g. rice noodles
1 litre water
1 tablesp. miso
½ teasp. Celtic salt
100 g. tempeh, cut into small cubes

1. Fry the onions in the oil for a few minutes.
2. Place onions, water and vegetables in a pot and bring to boil.
3. Blend the miso with a little of the hot water and add to the pot.
4. Add tempeh, rice noodles and salt and cook for 10 minutes.

9. VEGETARIAN MAIN MEALS

Salads
Chunky Salad
This is a colourful blend of raw salad vegetables.
raw beetroot (peeled)

raw carrots
celery
raw asparagus
raw snow peas
radishes

1. Cut raw beetroot, carrots and celery into long strips.
2. Add raw snow peas and radishes.
3. Arrange on a flat glass plate. Decorate with parsley.

Chick Pea Salad
1 cup chick peas, soaked, rinsed and cooked
1 spring onion, chopped
1 stick celery, chopped
parsley, chopped
1 tablesp. cold-pressed olive oil
1 tablesp. lemon juice
¼ teasp. each cumin, turmeric and coriander
½ teasp. Celtic salt or Herbamare salt

Combine all ingredients. Add Celtic salt. Chill.
If available, use fresh coriander.

Tabouleh Salad
¼ cup burghul
2 tomatoes, finely chopped
1 spring onion finely chopped
½ cup parsley finely chopped
½ cup peeled, chopped cucumber
¼ cup finely chopped fresh coriander
¼ teasp. dry dill
¼ teasp. sweet paprika
¼ teasp. Celtic salt
1 dessertsp. lemon juice
1 dessertsp. cold-pressed olive oil

1. Soak burghul in warm water for 10 minutes.
2. Drain and spread out on absorbent paper.

3. Combine all ingredients in a bowl and mix gently.
4. Serve with salad vegetables.
This dish is similar to rice salad but has a nuttier texture.

Rice Salad
2 cups cooked brown rice
1 stick of celery, finely chopped
½ cup sunflower seeds
½ cup sprouted mung beans
½ cup grated carrot
¼ cup finely chopped capsicum
½ teasp. Celtic salt
1 tablesp. lemon juice
1 dessertsp. cold-pressed olive oil

1. Combine all ingredients with cooled rice.
2. Mix in the lemon juice and oil.
For coarse grain Celtic salt, use a mortar and pestle to make it fine

Rice and avocado salad
2 cups cooked, cold brown rice
1 clove garlic, crushed
1 ripe avocado, chopped
2 tablesp. sunflower seeds
3 tomatoes, chopped
½ teasp. Celtic salt
½ teasp. sweet paprika
1 dessertsp. lemon juice
1 dessertsp. olive oil
1 tablesp. chopped parsley

1. Combine all ingredients with cooled rice.
2. Mix in the lemon juice and oil.
For coarse grain Celtic salt, use a mortar and pestle to make it fine.
Spring onion, red salad onion or chives may be substituted for garlic.

Potato Salad
4 potatoes, chopped into cubes

¼ cup chopped mint
¼ cup chopped parsley
¼ cup chopped chives
2 tablesp. natural organic yoghurt
½ teasp. Celtic salt
¼ teasp. sweet paprika

1. Steam potato cubes until cooked, but not soft, (about 5-10 minutes).
2. Cool potato and add greens.
3. Stir into the yoghurt, Celtic salt and sweet paprika.
4. Add yoghurt to other ingredients and stir gently.

For coarse grain Celtic salt, use a mortar and pestle to make it fine.

Avocado Salad
1 ripe avocado
2 tablesp. chopped walnuts, hazelnuts or macadamia nuts
2 sticks celery, diced
1 tablesp. natural yoghurt
¼ teasp. sweet paprika
¼ teasp. Celtic salt

1. Mash avocado on a bowl.
2. Stir in yoghurt, paprika, salt, nuts and celery
3. Serve on crisp lettuce leaves.

For coarse grain Celtic salt, use a mortar and pestle to make it fine.

Coleslaw
2 medium carrots, grated
1 stick celery, chopped fine
¼ salad onion, chopped
250 g. cabbage, shredded
1 tablesp. lemon juice
1 teasp. honey
½ cup walnuts, chopped

Prepare vegetables. Place them in a bowl and toss with lemon and honey.
If preferred, use 'Mayonnaise' from Salad dressings and dips section, instead of the lemon juice and honey.

For coarse grain Celtic salt, use a mortar and pestle to make it fine.

Mung Bean Salad
225 g. sprouted mung beans
225 g. carrots, cut into sticks
1 stick celery, chopped
1 capsicum
30 g. walnuts or pine nuts
30 g. sesame seeds
1 tablesp. olive oil
1 dessertsp. lemon juice
1 dessertsp. Tamari
Combine all ingredients. Toss.

Spinach-Avocado salad
225 g. (5 cups) spinach, torn into pieces
1 ripe avocado, finely chopped
2 tomatoes, cut into wedges
30 g. sunflower seeds
Combine all ingredients. Toss.

Bean Salad
1 tin white beans or 3-bean mix, rinsed
1 stick celery
½ salad onion, chopped
1 spring onion, chopped
1 tablesp. chives
1 tablesp. parsley
1 cup green beans, chopped
1 piece capsicum, chopped
1 tomato, chopped
1 tablesp. olive oil
1 dessertsp. lemon juice
½ teasp. sweet paprika
¼ teasp. Celtic salt
Combine all ingredients. Toss.

Lentil Salad
1 cups green lentils, soaked and rinsed
3 cups water
1 teasp. Celtic salt
½ teasp. each cumin and turmeric
1 dessertsp. olive oil
1 spring onion
1 tablesp. chopped chives
1 tablesp. chopped parsley
1 tablesp. fresh coriander, chopped
½ cup finely chopped carrot
1 stick celery, chopped

1. Boil lentils in water until cooked, but not too soft. (about 25 minutes).
2. Drain off any excess water.
3. Add salt, cumin and turmeric and stir in while lentils are hot. Allow to cool.
4. Mix in all other ingredients.

Beetroot Salad
1 raw beetroot
1 carrot
1 stick celery
¼ red salad onion or some chopped chives
fresh parsley
½ teasp. Celtic salt
1 dessertsp. lemon juice
1 teasp. honey

1. Grate carrot and beetroot fairly coarsely.
2. Add chopped celery and onion.
3. Add lemon juice, salt and honey. Toss.
Alternative method: Place all ingredients in food processor and chop.

VEGETABLE DISHES

Home-Made Tomato and Vegetable Puree
400 g. tin tomatoes or equivalent in freshly cooked tomatoes

1 tablesp. tomato paste
1 onion
1 stick celery
1 small zucchini
1 tablesp. parsley
½ teasp. each of dried basil, thyme and oregano
1 teasp. Celtic salt

Blend all ingredients together in blender and then simmer on stove for about 15 minutes.

Ratatouille

1 onion, chopped
1 cup chopped eggplant
1 cup chopped zucchini
1 stick chopped celery
1 tablesp. chopped parsley
400 g. tin tomatoes, or equivalent in fresh
1 dessertsp. cold-pressed olive oil
1 dessertsp. miso or vegetable stock

1. Saute onion in olive oil.
2. Stir in other vegetables except for tomatoes and continue to stir-fry for a minute.
3. Dissolve the miso or stock cube with a little boiling water.
4. Add this stock to the vegetables and simmer until eggplant is cooked.
5. Lastly add tomatoes and stir in very gently.
6. Serve with brown rice.

Curried Vegetables and Brown Rice

1 onion, chopped
1 dessertsp. olive oil
1 cup diced pumpkin
1 mixed vegetables – carrot, sweet potato, celery, zucchini
1 teasp. turmeric
1 chopped fresh tomato
½ teasp. coriander, or some fresh coriander
½ teasp. cumin

¼ cup sultanas
½ teasp. Celtic salt
1 cup water

1. Saute onion in olive oil.
2. Add all other ingredients and simmer for 20 minutes.
3. Serve over brown rice. Add some nuts or pepitas for protein.

Nut Stir-Fry
2 dessertsp. olive oil
1 onion, chopped
1 clove garlic, crushed
1 tomato, chopped
1 capsicum, sliced
2 cups green beans
50 g. almonds split into halves, or cashews
1 ripe avocado
½ teasp. celtic salt
½ teasp. turmeric
½ cup water

Cooked Brown Rice
1. Lightly pan-fry nuts in 1 dessertsp. olive oil. Transfer to a dish and set aside for garnish.
2. Saute onion and garlic in 1 dessertsp. olive oil.
3. Add water, green beans, onions, tomato, capsicum, salt and turmeric and stir-fry for 5 minutes.
4. Serve over cooked brown rice.
5. Garnish with avocado and nuts.

Baked Potato Chips
1. Peel potatoes and dry them.
2. Cut into chip shapes or wedges.
3. Place chips on a wire rack. A cake cooling rack will do.
4. Bake in the oven at 180 degrees C.

No oil is needed for cooking chips to brown. However chips may be brushed lightly with cold-pressed olive oil if desired.

Chinese Stir-Fry

1 chopped onion
selection of chopped vegetables
mung bean sprouts
1 cup water
1 dessertsp. cold-pressed olive oil
1 teasp. miso or vegetable stock cube
1 tablesp. tamari or kelp sauce
1 cup chopped tempeh, or 2 boiled eggs
pumpkin seeds, sunflower seeds, almonds or cashews

1. Using a wok or large frying pan, saute onion in olive oil.
2. Stir in favourite chopped vegetables, e.g. celery, carrot, bok choy, broccoli, zucchini, cabbage, capsicum, green beans and sprouts.
3. Add chopped tempeh. Continue to stir.
4. Add water, miso or stock cube, tamari or kelp sauce. Simmer for 5 minutes, stirring occasionally.
5. Sprinkle with sunflower seeds pumpkin seeds or almonds. Add chopped egg if desired.
6. Serve with wholegrain rice.
Dried seaweed, boiled as directed on packet, can be added to stir-fry dishes.

Thai Style Stir-Fried Vegetables

1 tablesp. olive oil
100 g. snow peas
100 g. broccoli or cauliflower
100 g. cabbage
1 carrot
1 stick celery
½ capsicum
1 onion
1 cup shelled peas
200g. tin coconut milk
1 piece fresh ginger
lemon grass, dried or freshly chopped
1 tablesp. Kelpamare sauce or Tamari
1 teasp. cornflour mixed with ½ cup water

1. Stir fry onion in olive oil.
2. Add other vegetables and continue to stir-fry for 30 seconds.
3. Add all other ingredients and cook for 5 minutes.
4. Serve with coconut brown rice. (Stir in some coconut oil to the rice before serving).
Add nuts or pepitas for protein.

Tomato and Beans with Greens

400 g. tin tomatoes
1 onion
2 cups cooked haricot beans
parsley and basil
2 cups of green vegetables

1. Blend tomatoes and onion. Place in saucepan and simmer 5 minutes.
2. Add cooked haricot beans.
3. Add raw green vegetables.
4. Simmer for a further 2 minutes, so that the vegetables are crisp and retain nutrition.

Cauliflower in White Sauce

1 cauliflower, broken into pieces and lightly steamed
½ onion
2 cups water
1 tablesp. organic natural yoghurt
2 tablesp. brown rice flour
½ onion
2 tablesp. parsley
1 clove garlic
1 teasp. Celtic salt
¼ teasp. sweet paprika
sesame seeds or breadcrumbs made from 'good bread'

1. Arrange cauliflower to fill the base of a casserole dish.
2. Blend all other ingredients in a blender.
3. Pour blended mixture into a saucepan and make a white sauce by stirring over the heat until boiling.
4. Pour sauce over cauliflower.

5. Sprinkle with sesame seeds or breadcrumbs.
6. Bake in a moderate oven for 20 minutes.

Sweet Potato au Gratin

3 sweet potatoes
3 potatoes
1 clove garlic
1 teasp. Celtic salt
1 cup cooked peas
½ cup arrowroot or brown rice flour
100 g. cashews
4 cups water

1. Steam vegetables.
2. Blend cashews, flour, salt and garlic in water.
3. Pour over drained vegetables.
4. Add peas and bake for 20 minutes at 200 degrees C.

Stews, Casseroles and Hot Pots

Moussaka

1 tablesp. cold-pressed olive oil
1 onion, chopped or grated
1 clove garlic, crushed (optional)
400 g. tin tomatoes
1 stick celery
1 teasp. dried basil
1 medium eggplants, sliced
2 cups brown or green lentils, soaked, rinsed
2 teasp. Celtic salt
Quantity of Savoury Cashew Spread

1. Cut eggplant into slices and bake at 180 degrees C. for 15 minutes, or pan-fry in a little olive oil.
2. Blend tomatoes and onion.
3. Drain lentils and mix with blended tomato and onion. Add basil, chopped celery and salt. Pour into casserole dish.
4. Arrange eggplant slices on top of lentil and tomato mixture.

5. For the topping, use 'Savoury Cashew Spread' *(see Cheese Substitutes section).*
6. Bake at 180 degrees C for 30 minutes.

2 cups cooked red kidney beans may be substituted for lentils.

Eggplant Italian

2 potatoes, steamed and diced
1 eggplant, diced
1 zucchini, diced
3 tomatoes, chopped
1 onion, grated
2 tablesp. brown rice flour
½ teasp. each dried basil and oregano (or equivalent in fresh herbs)
1 teasp. tamari or kelp sauce
3 tablesp. wheatgerm or sesame seeds
½ teasp. Celtic salt

1. Saute the onion, egg plant, zucchini, tomato in a little olive oil.
2. Stir in the flour, herbs, salt and water and cook for one minute.
3. Place cooked potatoes in a casserole dish.
5. Spoon the vegetable sauce mixture over the potatoes.
6. Sprinkle wheat germ or sesame seeds.
7. Bake in moderate oven without lid for 15 minutes.

Mexican Beans

2 cups red kidney beans
1½ litres water
400 g. tin tomatoes
1 tablesp. tomato paste
1 onion
½ capsicum
1 teasp. dried basil
½ teasp. oregano
1 teasp. sweet paprika
1 tablesp. parsley
1 clove garlic
1 bay leaf
½ teasp. cumin
2 teasp. salt

1. Soak, rinse and cook beans in water.
2. Place all other ingredients except for beans in blender and blend.
3. Place blended mixture in saucepan with cooked beans. Bring to boil and simmer 15-20 minutes.

Serve over rice, or in a scooped out baked potato in jacket. (Mash the scooped out potato and put it on top.) Alternatively, serve with tortillas. *(See next recipe.)* Goes well with mushrooms and sweet corn.

Mexican Tortilla

1½ cups plain flour
1 cup maize meal
1 cup water

1. Mix the flour and meal together with water. Use just enough water to make a firm dough.
2. Knead and roll out as pastry, (not too thin).
3. Cook tortillas in electric fry pan on high heat in a similar way to pancakes. Flip when one bottom side is cooked.
4. To keep warm, wrap in baking paper and place in a casserole dish with lid on, in a warm oven.

This recipe also works well in a waffle maker.

Bean and Vegetable Hot Pot

1 cup red kidney beans
1 cup Lima beans
½ cup red lentils
1 litre water
2 tablesp. tomato paste
400 g. tin tomatoes
1 onion
1 teasp. miso or natural vegetable cube
½ teasp. Celtic salt
2 cups vegetables diced and steamed.

1. Soak, rinse and cook dried beans and lentils altogether in water. Drain.
2. Blend tomatoes and onion in blender.
3. Place cooked beans, lentils, tomato paste, blended tomato and onion and seasonings together in saucepan.

4. Add diced, steamed vegetables of your choice. Serve in large pasta dishes.

Pumpkin Hot Pot
4 cups diced pumpkin
1 onion, chopped or grated
2 carrots
1 zucchini
1 cup diced celery
½ diced capsicum
400 g. tin tomatoes, roughly chopped
1 teasp. Celtic salt
1 teasp. honey
1 teasp. tomato paste
2 bay leaves
¼ teasp. sweet paprika

1. Steam pumpkin, carrot, celery and zucchini for 5 minutes.
2. Saute onion and capsicum in olive oil.
3. Mix all ingredients together in casserole dish. Bake with lid on for 20 minutes.

Haricot Beans in Tomato Sauce
2 cups haricot beans
750 ml. water
1 dessertsp. tomato paste
400 g. tin tomatoes
1 onion
2 teasp. Celtic salt
Italian herbs

1. Soak, rinse and cook beans in 750 ml water. Drain.
2. Blend tomatoes, tomato paste, onion Celtic salt and herbs in a blender.
3. Simmer in large saucepan for 15 minutes.
This is a good substitute for tinned baked beans. Serve with salad.

Spiced Chick Peas
2 cups chickpeas, soaked and rinsed
1 litre water

1 medium onion
1 clove garlic
1 tablesp. olive oil
1 teasp. cumin seeds
1 teasp. dried corriander or 2 tablsp. fresh corriander
1 teasp. ground turmeric
½ teasp. sweet paprika
2 teasp. Celtic salt
1 tablesp. tomato paste
200 g. chopped vegetables - pumpkin, carrot, sweet potato

1. Cook chick peas in water for 30 minutes. Drain and save 1cup liquid.
2. Stir-fry chopped onion and garlic in olive oil in a pan.
3. Add to pan: spices, salt, tomato paste, chopped vegetables and saved liquid. Stir over heat for 30 seconds.
4. Place this mixture in saucepan with chickpeas and simmer with lid on for 20 minutes, stirring occasionally.
5. Sprinkle with chopped fresh parsley.

Red Lentil Dahl

2 cups red lentils
1 litre water
½ teasp. cumin
¼ teasp. cardamom
½ teasp. coriander, or handful fresh coriander
1 teasp. turmeric
1 clove garlic
1 onion
1 tablesp. tomato paste
2 teasp. Celtic salt

1. Soak and rinse lentils.
2. Cook lentils in water in a large saucepan until soft.
3. Stir-fry onion and garlic in a little water or olive oil.
4. Add onion, tomato paste, spices and salt to the lentils. Cook for another 5-10 minutes.

For an Italian flavour, substitute the herbs and spices for basil, oregano and thyme.

Split Pea Dahl
2 cups yellow split peas
½ cup red lentils
800 ml. water
1 onion
1 clove garlic, crushed
1 teasp. coriander or 2 tablesp. fresh
1 teasp. turmeric
1 teasp. ground cumin seeds
1 teasp. ground mustard seeds
400 g. tin tomatoes
½ capsicum
1 tablesp. olive oil
2 teasp. Celtic salt

1. Soak and rinse split peas and lentils. Cook in water in large saucepan until soft.
2. Stir-fry chopped onion, garlic and mustard seeds in olive oil in a pan.
3. Add to pan, chopped capsicum, herbs and spices and continue to stir over heat for a few minutes.
4. Mix ingredients from pan to the split peas in the saucepan. Add salt and tomatoes and simmer for another 10 minutes.
Seeds may be ground with a mortar and pestle.

Layered Vegetable Casserole
3 cups vegetables, chopped and steamed
e.g. potato, carrot, celery, zucchini, broccoli, peas or beans
1 cup uncooked pasta, e.g. wholemeal, rice or corn pasta
400 g. tin tomatoes
1 tablesp. tomato paste
1 onion
½ capsicum
basil and parsley
1 natural vegetable stock cube
2 slices 'good bread', crumbed
½ teasp. Celtic salt
¼ teasp. sweet paprika
2 tablesp. cornflour or brown rice flour

1. Steam the vegetables.
2. Boil pasta for time specified on packet. Drain and place aside.
3. Blend together in a blender: tomatoes, tomato paste, onion, capsicum, basil, parsley and stock cube.
4. Mix cooked pasta with blended mixture in a casserole dish, making the first layer.
5. Place steamed potatoes and carrots on top of pasta, then greens. This forms the second layer.
6. Make a white sauce from 2 tablesp. cornflour or brown rice flour, 2 cups of cold water and half a stock cube. Whisk while bringing to boil. Pour white sauce over top of vegetables.
7. Bake casserole with a lid for about 30 minutes. Remove lid, sprinkle with breadcrumbs and bake for a few more minutes.

Pasta and Pizza
Use wholemeal pasta, rice or corn pasta

Lentil Bolognaise
2 cups brown, green or red lentils, soaked and rinsed
1 litre water
1 onion
400 g. tin tomatoes
1 tablesp. tomato paste
1 teasp. dried Italian herbs (basil, oregano, thyme)
1 teasp. Celtic salt

1. Cook lentils in water in a large saucepan.
2. Blend all other ingredients in blender.
3. Add blended ingredients to cooked lentils and cook for half an hour. Add salt.

This sauce can be poured over pasta for a kind of 'spaghetti bolognaise'. It can also be used as the base layer for a lentil and vegetable lasagne.
For a curry flavour, substitute Italian herbs with cumin, turmeric and coriander.

Lentil Lasagne
quantity of 'Lentil Bolognaise' *(previous recipe)*
pasta sheets (whole wheat, corn or rice pasta)

quantity of 'Savoury Cashew Spread' (see Butter, Cream and Cheese substututes)

1. Boil pasta for 5 minutes. To cool quickly, transfer to a bowl of cold water. Drain.
2. Lay half of the pasta sheets at the bottom of a square or rectangular oven-proof dish.
3. Spoon on 'Lentil Bolognaise' mixture.
4. Place the rest of the pasta sheets on top.
5. Spoon the 'Savoury Cashew Spread' over the pasta sheets.
6. Bake at 180 degrees C for 15–20 minutes.

Vegetable Lasagne
6 lasagne sheets
400 g. tin tomatoes, chopped
1 tablesp. tomato paste
basil, oregano and thyme (dried or fresh)
1 teasp. Celtic salt and/or vegetable stock cube
1 onion, chopped
1 tablesp. olive oil
3 cups chopped, vegetables (various)
quantity of Savoury Cashew Spread (See Butter, Cream and Cheese Substitutes)

1. Lightly steam the vegetables.
2. Boil lasagne sheets in a large saucepan for 5 minutes. Pour off the boiling water and stand lasagne sheets in cold water.
3. In a frying pan, saute onion in olive oil. Add tomatoes, herbs, salt and tomato paste. Then gently stir in steamed vegetables.
4. Place half of the lasagne sheets in a square or rectangular oven-proof dish, to form the bottom layer.
5. Spoon on steamed vegetable mixture.
6. Place another layer of the remaining pasta on top.
7. Spoon the 'Savoury Cashew Spread' over the pasta sheets.
8. Bake in a moderate oven 15-20 minutes.

Pesto with Pasta
1 cup fresh basil (10-12 leaves)

50 g. pine nuts
1 dessertsp. cold-pressed olive oil
½ teasp. Celtic salt
1 tablesp. lemon juice
¼ teasp. sweet paprika
2 tablesp. water

1. Blend all ingredients in food processor.
2. Serve over hot pasta.

Creamy Pasta
2 cups uncooked tubular pasta
For sauce:
1 tablesp. tahini
2 cups water
2 tablesp. brown rice flour or maize flour
½ onion
2 tablesp parsley
1 cup chopped celery
1 clove garlic
1 teasp. Celtic salt
½ teasp. sweet paprika

1. Boil pasta according to directions on packet, drain and place in an oven-proof dish.
2. Place all other ingredients in the blender and blend.
3. Pour blended mixture into a saucepan and make it into a sauce by stirring over the heat until it comes to the boil.
4. Pour sauce over drained pasta.
5. Sprinkle with nuts, sesame seeds or breadcrumbs and bake in a moderate oven 20 minutes.
Serve with fresh parsley and basil, as a complement to a salad.

Vegetable Pasta Sauce
1 small cauliflower, cut in pieces
100 g. mushrooms
1 stick celery, diced
1 onion, chopped

1 tablesp. olive oil
½ capsicum, diced
2 cups water
1 tablesp. rice flour or cornflour
1 teasp. Celtic salt
½ teasp. sweet paprika

1. In wok, or electric fry-pan, or large saucepan, saute onion in olive oil.
2. Add all the vegetables and 1 cup water. Stir, bring to boil and simmer for 5 minutes, with lid on.
3. Mix rice flour in 1 cup water, and add. Stir while bringing to boil.
4. Serve over fettuccine pasta.

Mushroom Pasta Sauce
2 cups mushrooms, sliced
1 onion, chopped
1 cup water
1 teasp. Celtic salt
¼ teasp. grated nutmeg
1 teasp. grated lemon rind
1 dessertsp. cold-pressed olive oil
1 dessertsp. rice flour or cornflour

1. Stir fry onion in olive oil. Add mushrooms and continue to stir.
2. Whisk rice flour with water and add. Bring to boil while stirring.
3. Add lemon rind and nutmeg. Continue to stir for a few minutes.
4. Serve over fettuccine pasta.

Pizza Base:
Wholemeal pita bread

Topping:
quantity tomato paste/tomato puree
quantity Savoury Cashew Spread (Refer to 'Butter, Cream and Cheese Substitutes')
1 teasp. dried Italian herbs (basil, oregano and thyme)
favourite vegetable toppings e.g, mushrooms, celery, tomato, chives, capsicum, zucchini, pine nuts

1. Spread the tomato paste over pita bread.
2. Spread 'Savoury Cashew Spread' generously over tomato paste.
3. Add chopped or sliced vegetables. Sprinkle with pine nuts.
4. Bake 15-20 minutes in a moderate oven.

BURGERS, PANCAKES AND VEGIE-LOAVES

Vegie Burgers

2 cups steamed pumpkin, sweet potato or carrot
1 cup steamed potato
1 stick celery, finely chopped
1 onion, chopped or grated
1 clove garlic
1 tablesp. miso or 2 tablesp. tamari
1 tablesp. tahini
1 beaten egg
parsley and basil
½ cup rice flour
1 dessertsp. tomato paste/tomato puree
1 cup breadcrumbs (from 'good' bread)

1. Mash the vegetables.
2. Add all other ingredients except for flour and breadcrumbs.
3. Mix thoroughly, lastly mixing in flour and breadcrumbs.
4. Form burgers. Bake in oven or fry with a little olive oil in fry pan. If frying, turn three times.

Curried Vegie-Burgers

½ cup mashed pumpkin or sweet potato
1 cup mashed potato
2 cups grated carrot
2 sticks celery
½ zucchini
2 tablesp. parsley
2 tablesp. tahini
1 teasp. Celtic salt
2 tablesp. rice flour
1 teasp. mild curry powder

1 cup wheat germ

1. Combine all ingredients in food processor.
2. Place in scoops in an oven-proof dish. Flatten like pancakes.
3. Bake in moderate oven for about 15 minutes.

Alternatively make as burgers in fry-pan, using a little olive. For fry-pan method, turn three times.

Lentil Burgers
3 cups cooked, drained brown lentils
1 cup mashed potato
1 cup mashed pumpkin and carrot
½ cup sesame seeds
½ cup ground almonds
½ cup grated carrot
1 small onion, grated
1 tablesp. kelp sauce or tamari
1 teasp. Celtic salt
2 tablesp. buckwheat or brown rice flour

1. Combine all ingredients and mix well.
2. Place in scoops in an oven-proof dish. Flatten like pancakes.
3. Bake in moderate oven for about 20 minutes

Alternatively make as burgers in electric fry-pan, using a little olive. For fry-pan method, turn three times.

Quinoa Burgers
1 cup quinoa cooked in 2 cups water
1 cup mashed potato
1 tablesp. tahini
1 teasp. Celtic salt
½ cup grated carrot
1 onion, chopped or grated
½ cup cooked corn
parsley and favourite fresh herbs

1. Drain quinoa and set aside.
2. Mix all other ingredients in a bowl.

3. Add quinoa and make into patties.
4. Bake in moderate oven for 20 minutes.
Alternatively make as burgers in electric fry-pan, using a little olive oil. For fry-pan method, turn three times.
Quinoa is a grain similar to millet. Very nutritious!

Tempeh Balls

300 g. mashed tempeh
1 small grated onion
¼ cup rice milk
2 slices bread
2 tablesp. rice flour
2 tablesp. wheat germ
2 tablesp. chopped parsley
1 tablesp kelp sauce or tamari
½ vegetable stock cube dissolved in water

1. Grate the bread into fine crumbs.
2. Grate the onion.
3. Add all other ingredients and mix together.
4. Mould into balls.
5. Bake in moderate oven 25 minutes, or shallow-fry in olive oil.

Tempeh balls can be use instead of meatballs in a thick soup such as minestrone.

Falafel

1 cup chick peas, soaked and cooked
1 onion
1 cup various steamed vegetables (include pumpkin, sweet potato or potato)
parsley & basil
2 tablesp. buckwheat flour
½ teasp. sweet paprika
1 teasp. Celtic salt
½ cup water

1. Place all ingredients in food processor and blend together. Add more water if necessary.
2. Scoop by the spoonful, like pancakes, into an oven-proof dish.

3. Bake in a moderate oven 20 minutes.

Alternatively make as burgers in electric fry-pan, using a little olive oil. For fry-pan method, turn three times.

Spinach Pancakes
4 cups spinach
2 tablesp. buckwheat flour
1 dessertsp. cornflour
1 tablesp. brown rice flour
1 egg
¾ cup rice milk
1 teasp. tamari or kelp sauce

1. Steam spinach and mix with all other ingredients.
2. Grease base of fry pan with cold-pressed olive oil.
3. Spoon pancake mixture into hot fry pan. Turn when ready.

Corn Fritters
1 cup flour e.g. buckwheat flour
1 egg
1 cup cooked corn
½ teasp. Celtic salt
1 tablesp. rice milk

1. Whisk all ingredients together except for corn.
2. Add corn to the mixture and stir.
3. Grease electric fry-pan with cold-pressed olive oil.
4. Drop by spoonful and turn when ready.

Potato and Corn Patties
2 cups mashed potato
1½ cups cooked corn kernels
1 tablesp. rice milk or water
1 egg white
¼ teasp. sweet paprika
¼ cup chives
breadcrumbs from 'good bread'

1. Mash potato with rice milk and Celtic salt.
2. Mix all ingredients together and make patties.
3. Roll in breadcrumbs and bake in a moderate oven for about 20 minutes, or make patties and fry in a little olive oil.

Tempeh Vegie Loaf

375 g. tempeh
2 tablsp. tamari
2 tablesp. tahini or 2 beaten eggs
1 onion, chopped or grated
1 cup grated carrot
chopped celery, capsicum and zucchini as desired
½ cup chopped parsley
2 cloves garlic, crushed
½ teasp. dried sweet basil, or fresh basil
3 cups breadcrumbs made from 'good' bread, or 2 cups cooked brown rice

1. Mash tempeh with a fork and mix thoroughly with the tamari.
2. Add all other ingredients and mix thoroughly.
3. Lightly oil a loaf-tin or casserole dish, packing mixture down firmly.
4. Bake at 180 degrees C for 45 - 50 minutes.

Nut Burgers

1 onion
½ teasp. dried herbs
2 slices 'good' bread
1 dessertsp. savoury yeast flakes, or ½ stock cube
1 dessertsp kelp sauce or tamari
½ small zucchini (100 g.) or 1 stick celery
1½ cups sunflower seeds or nuts
¼ cup water

1. Grind seeds or nuts in food processor.
2. Break bread into pieces. Combine all ingredients in food processor and blend.
3. Drop spoonfuls of the mixture into an electric fry-pan greased with olive oil. Turn after a few minutes. Cook and turn twice more.

Note: Savoury yeast flakes are made from torula yeast, which is non-living and does not cause candida.

Oatmeal-Almond Loaf

½ cup ground almonds
1 cup hot water
½ cup celery, chopped
1 teasp. Celtic salt
1 teasp. mixed herbs or fresh herbs
½ cup water
½ cup ground sunflower seeds or cashews
1 cup rolled oats
1 onion, chopped
1 cup bread crumbs
½ cup chick peas, soaked and rinsed

1. Blend chick peas with 1 cup water.
2. Combine with hot water, the oats, onion, bread crumbs, celery, salt, herbs, almonds and sunflower seeds.
3. Add blended chick peas and stir.
4. Allow to stand for a few minutes.
5. Press into loaf shaped baking dish. Bake at 180 degrees C for 50 minutes.

GRAINS

Quinoa Stuffed Capsicum

1 cup quinoa cooked in 2 cups water
4 to 6 medium capsicums
1 onion, chopped or grated
150 g. fresh mushrooms, sliced
400 g. tin tomatoes
1 clove garlic
1 teasp. Celtic salt
½ teasp. sweet paprika
1 dessertsp. olive oil
breadcrumbs

1. Cook quinoa and set aside.
2. Cut capsicums in half and remove seeds.
3. Steam capsicums until soft but not limp.
4. Saute onion and crushed garlic in olive oil.

5. Combine all ingredients except for quinoa and capsicums. Reserve half of the tomato juice. Stir-fry for 5 minutes.
6. Fold in quinoa.
7. Place capsicums in a baking dish and stuff with quinoa mixture. This will take about half the mixture.
8. Thin remainder with reserved juice and pour around capsicums. Sprinkle breadcrumbs over top. Sprinkle a little fine Celtic salt over breadcrumbs.
9. Bake in a moderate oven for 30 minutes.

Millet Bake

2 cups millet, cooked and drained
½ teasp. Celtic salt
400 g. tin tomatoes
1 stick celery
parsley and fresh basil, chopped finely
1 onion, chopped
1 capsicum, chopped
1 tablesp. olive oil
1 tablesp. tahini
1 egg

1. Saute onion in olive oil.
2. Mix all ingredients together.
3. Pour into pie dish and sprinkle with fresh breadcrumbs and slivered almonds. Sprinkle with fine Celtic salt.
4. Bake in a moderate oven 30 minutes.

Barley and Zucchini Bake

2 cups cooked barley, (pearled or unpearled)
2 medium onions, chopped
1 clove garlic
4-6 small zucchinis, sliced
200 g. mushrooms, sliced
1 cup chopped eggplant
½ teasp. Celtic salt dissolved in 1 tablesp. boiling water
2 tablesp. tahini
1 tablesp. cold-pressed olive oil

1. Saute onion and garlic in olive oil. Continue to stir-fry, adding eggplant and zucchini. Lastly add sliced mushrooms and cook slightly.
2. Mix pan-fried vegetables with cooked barley, salted water and tahini.
3. Place mixture in an oven-proof dish and bake at 180 degrees C. for 30 minutes.

Buckwheat and mushrooms

1 cup uncooked cooked buckwheat kernels
1 onion
1 clove garlic
2 sliced tomatoes
1 tablesp. olive oil
200 g. mushrooms
½ teasp. sweet paprika
½ teasp. Celtic salt
1 tablesp. Tamari

1. Boil buckwheat in water for about 15 minutes, until grains are soft.
2. Pan-fry onion and garlic in olive oil. Add mushrooms and tomato and stir-fry for another minute.
3. Combine pan-fried ingredients, salt, tomato paste and Tamari with buckwheat. Stir gently and heat through.

Pies and Pastries

Nut Pastry

½ cup wholemeal flour
½ cup buckwheat flour
½ cup barley or millet flour
½ cup ground almonds or cashews
½ cup water
1 dessertsp. cold-pressed olive oil

1. Process nuts in food processor until fine.
2. Add flours and olive oil.
3. Add enough water while blending to make a firm dough.
4. Chill and roll out.

This recipe will also work with all wheat-free flours.

Potato Pastry
1 cup flour
½ cup mashed potato
rice milk or water to mix.

1. Combine all ingredients, adding enough water or milk to make a dough.
2. Chill and roll out.
For savoury dishes, this pastry can be used as an alternative to nut pastry.

Shepherd's Pie
2 cups brown or green lentils, soaked, rinsed and cooked
1 onion (chopped or grated)
1 vegetable stock cube
2 tablesp. tomato paste
½ teasp. Celtic salt.
quantity mashed potato

1. Drain lentils reserving 1cup liquid.
2. Stir in tomato paste, onion, salt, stock cube and reserved liquid. Simmer for about 10 minutes.
3. Pour into casserole dish.
4. Place mashed potato on top.
5. Bake in a moderate oven for 30 minutes.

Lentil Pie
Quantity 'Nut Pastry'
2 cups brown or green lentils, soaked, rinsed and cooked
1 onion (chopped or grated)
1 vegetable stock cube
2 tablesp. tomato paste
½ teasp. Celtic salt.

1. Drain cooked lentils reserving 1cup liquid.
2. Stir in tomato paste, onion, salt, stock cube and reserved liquid. Simmer for about 10 minutes.
3. Divide nut pastry in two. Roll out and line a pie dish. Bake pastry shell for 5-10 minutes.
4. Spoon in lentils. Top with pastry.

5. Bake in a moderate oven for 25 minutes.

Mushroom and Lentil Pie
quantity of 'Nut Pastry'
2 dessertsp. brown or green lentils
1 dessertsp. red lentils
1 large onion, chopped or grated
1 tablesp. cold-pressed olive oil
1 stick celery, finely chopped
½ vegetable stock cube
½ teasp. mixed dried herbs, or fresh
2 cups mushrooms, sliced
1 cup diced eggplant
½ cup cooked peas
½ medium carrot, finely diced
1 tablesp. kelp sauce or tamari
¼ teasp. Celtic salt
1 dessertsp. rice flour or corn flour

1. Soak and cook lentils. Drain, reserving ½ cup liquid.
2. Prepare pie base and bake 10 minutes.
3. Add carrot and celery, stock cube, salt and kelp sauce to lentils and ½ cup liquid.
4. Simmer for a few minutes.
5. Thicken with rice flour or corn flour.
6. Stir fry onion, mushrooms, eggplant in 1 tablesp. cold-pressed olive oil.
7. Add onion, mushrooms and eggplant to lentil mixture. Add cooked peas. Stir.
8. Pour filling into pie base and add top pastry. Bake in a moderate oven 30 minutes.

Arame Rolls
1 large onion
1 clove garlic
1 large carrot
1 medium parsnip
½ cup parsley
1 cup cooked brown rice

1½ cups tempeh
1 tablesp. dried arame
1 tablesp. tamari sauce (or kelp sauce)
1 quantity of nut pastry or pita bread

1. Boil arame for 15 minutes. Drain.
2. Place all ingredients, except for arame and rice, in food processor and blend.
3. Place blended mixture, in a bowl.
4. Stir in arame and rice. This forms the filling.
5. Roll out pastry, and place filling into pastry as if you were making sausage rolls. Make a long roll which can be cut into smaller segments. Alternatively make as a pie, or fill pita bread pockets.
6. Bake in moderate oven 30 minutes.

Spring Rolls
quantity nut pastry
2 cups spring cabbage, slightly steamed
2 cups cooked brown rice
1 tablesp. tamari
½ teasp. Celtic salt

1. Combine all ingredients together in a bowl.
2. Bake in pastry rolls as for 'Arame Rolls'. (previous recipe)

Pumpkin Pasties
4 cups cooked pumpkin
2 cups cooked brown rice
1 onion, chopped
1 clove garlic
fresh coriander
quantity of nut pastry

1. Stir fry onion, garlic and coriander in a little water.
2. Add to cooked pumpkin and rice.
3. Make pastry and roll out. Cut round shapes about 15cm in diameter and make pasties.
4. Bake in moderate oven 30 minutes.

Spinach and Rice Pie

quantity of nut pastry
3 cups chopped spinach
1 onion, grated
1 cup cooked brown rice
1 small diced tomato
1 beaten egg
½ teasp. Celtic salt
1 tablesp. rice milk

1. Roll out pastry shell and bake in a moderate oven 5 minutes.
2. Water fry onion, tomato and spinach.
3. Mix other ingredients together and combine with vegetables.
4. Spoon into pastry case.
5. Bake in moderate oven for about 25 minutes.

Winter Pie

1 quantity of nut pastry
2 cups of 'winter' vegetables such as sweet potato, pumpkin, turnip, potato, carrot, parsnip
1 cup cooked chick peas
1 cup water
1 tablesp. rice flour
1 onion
1 stick celery
parsley and chives
1 teasp. Celtic salt
¼ teasp. sweet paprika

1. Dice and steam vegetables.
2. Prepare pastry shell and bake about 10 minutes.
3. Make white sauce in large saucepan, by whisking rice flour with water, continuing to whisk over heat until boiling.
4. Stir in chopped onion, celery, herbs, Celtic salt and sweet paprika.
5. Stir in cooked vegetables and chick peas.
6. Pour vegetable mixture into pastry shell.
7. Add a top layer of pastry.
8. Bake in moderate oven 25 minutes.

EGG DISHES

Zucchini Slice
1 onion
1 zucchini (160 g.)
1 stick celery
2 tablesp. parsley
1 cup cooked rice
4 eggs
1 teasp. Celtic salt
1 dessertsp. cold pressed olive oil
1 tablesp. rice flour

1. Place all ingredients in food processor and blend.
2. Pour into an ungreased oven proof dish. Bake 30-35 minutes.

Quiche
This makes two quiches, pie dish size 25 cm. diameter
1 quantity of nut pastry.
1 cup rice milk, or non-homogenised goat milk
1 onion
1 stick celery
parsley and chives
8 eggs
1 teas Celtic salt
½ teas sweet paprika
1 teasp. onion powder

1. Roll out pastry and line pie dishes. Bake in a moderate oven for 5 minutes.
2. Blend all ingredients in food processor, adding eggs last.
3. Pour egg mixture into pastry shells. Slice tomatoes and place on top. Bake 30 minutes.

Speedy Omelette
4 eggs
1 slice 'good bread', crumbed
½ teasp. Celtic salt

¼ grated onion
herbs as desired
1. Combine all ingredients.
2. Cook in fry-pan using a little cold-pressed olive oil.

10. FISH RECIPES

Fish oil is an excellent source of omega 3, but unfortunately most fish is contaminated with heavy metals, especially mercury. The following fish recipes should only be used if you have a guaranteed source of mercury-free fish. Small deep sea fish, (sardines), and Wild Alaskan Salmon are the safest. Farmed fish should be avoided. Also avoid any kind of smoked fish.
Note: For salted tinned salmon, do not add extra salt to recipes.

Baked Fish and Corn Casserole

210 g. tin of Alaskan wild salmon
2 cups cooked brown rice
1 cob sweet corn
1 cup chopped red and green capsicum
2 spring onions, chopped
½ teasp. Celtic salt
¼ teasp. sweet paprika
2 cups cold water
2 tablesp. rice flour
1 cup rye breadcrumbs and ½ cup flaked almonds

1. Remove corn from cob.
2. Make a white sauce from the water, rice flour, salt and paprika, stirring while bringing to the boil.
3. Stir all other ingredients into the sauce.
4. Place the mixture in a casserole dish and sprinkle with breadcrumbs and almonds.
5. Bake moderate oven 30 minutes.

Baked Fish and Potato Casserole

520 g. tin wild salmon
1 onion, grated or chopped finely
2 large potatoes
2 sticks celery chopped finely

1 piece chopped capsicum
1 tablesp. lemon juice
½ teasp. sweet paprika
1 egg

1. Steam the potatoes and mash with water.
2. Add all other ingredients to mashed potato.
3. Place into casserole dish and bake moderate oven for 30 minutes.

This mixture can be made into fish cakes. Roll in breadcrumbs and bake in moderate oven. For a finer mixture use a food processor.

Fish Soup

210 g. wild salmon
1 onion
½ cup diced celery
½ cup diced tomatoes
1 small diced zucchini
2 tablesp. flour (plain flour, buckwheat flour or rice flour)
½ teasp. Hungarian sweet paprika
¼ teasp. ground ginger or 1 piece fresh ginger
1 cup water
chopped parsley
¾ cup rolled oats
1½ cups water

1. Place onion, zucchini, celery and salt in water in a large saucepan. Bring to boil and simmer.
2. Add fish.
3. Mix the flour to a paste and add to saucepan, while stirring all the time. Simmer 5 minutes.
4. Add all other ingredients except for tomatoes. Simmer a further 4-5 minutes, stirring occasionally.
5. Lastly add tomatoes just before serving.

Fish Pasta Sauce

250 g. mushrooms
¾ cup tomato puree
½ onion, chopped
210 g. wild salmon

1 tablesp. chopped parsley
1 tablesp. fresh dill

1. Boil together in saucepan, tomato puree, onion, salt, parsley and dill.
2. Add mushrooms and simmer for a few minutes.
3. Add drained tinned fish. Continue to simmer a further 5 minutes.
4. Serve over pasta or brown rice.

Fish Cakes

210 g. wild salmon
1 cup mashed potato or cooked brown rice
1 egg
1 teasp. lemon juice
1 teasp. onion powder
breadcrumbs from 'good' bread

1. Mix all ingredients together except for the breadcrumbs.
2. Form balls from the fish mixture and roll in breadcrumbs. Bake in a moderate oven for about 15 minutes, or shallow fry in olive oil.

Salmon with Rice and Stir-Fried Vegetables

2 cups cooked brown rice
3 cups chopped vegetables (various)
1 dessertsp tamari mixed with ½ cup water
210 g. wild salmon

1. Stir fry vegetables for one minute. Add liquid.
2. Add rice and stir again.
3. Lastly add salmon. Don't stir vigorously. Just allow the salmon to heat through. Serve.

Fish, Potato and Rice Casserole

210 g. wild salmon
1 cup cooked brown rice
2 medium potatoes, cubed and steamed
1 egg, beaten
½ cup water
1 onion, chopped or grated

1 tablesp. olive oil
½ teasp. sweet paprika
parsley or dill, chopped
1 dessertsp. lemon juice
bread crumbs
almonds (split into halves)

1. Saute onion in olive oil.
2. Mix all ingredients together in a large bowl.
3. Spoon into casserole dish. Smooth out and sprinkle breadcrumbs and almonds on top.
4. Bake in moderate oven for 30 minutes.

11. FAST FOODS
You can make your own fast foods by preparing ahead.

Rice
Brown rice takes about 35 minutes to cook. This can be a problem if you are in a hurry. Brown rice is a staple food that can be prepared daily and kept in the fridge. Simply boil up a cup of rice first thing in the morning. Use a cooking mat for the hot plate to prevent burning or sticking to the bottom of the saucepan. Turn it off before you go out. (Turn off after about 30 minutes of cooking). It is now ready to be heated up any time in the day! Use kelp sauce, tamari or Celtic salt for seasoning. Serve with salad or vegetables. You can also use cooked rice for rice custard.
Brown rice will keep in a glass jar in the fridge for about 3 days.

Quick Stir Fry
Use a wok or electric fry-pan.
1. Saute onion in a little olive oil.
2. Add chopped vegetables. Continue to stir.
3. Add water and seasoning. (Use tamari, kelp sauce or Celtic salt)
4. Add cooked rice, continuing to stir for about 1 minute. The vegetables should be hot and crunchy. Do not over cook.

SOUP
Have soup on hand to quickly reheat. Store in glass jars in the fridge.

Beans
400 g. tin kidney beans or white beans
400 g. tin tomatoes
¼ vegetable stock cube
chopped celery, parsley and chives

1. Drain and rinse beans.
2. Dissolve stock cube with a little tomato juice in a saucepan over heat.
3. Add beans and the rest of the tomatoes. Stir over heat.

Toasted Sandwiches
Instead of butter and margarine, use 'Savoury Cashew Spread', *(see Butter, cream and cheese substitutes)*. The spread goes on the outside of the bread. Toast in an electric sandwich maker/jaffle maker. Delicious plain or with avocado and tomato filling.

Pizzas
Use pita bread. Spread with tomato paste and Savoury Cashew Spread as a replacement for cheese. Sprinkle with Italian herbs. Place under the grill for a minute.

12. SWEET TREATS FOR SPECIAL OCCASIONS
(Desserts, afternoon teas, slices, cakes and cookies)

Coconut used in these recipes may be replaced with sesame seeds or oat bran. To avoid the preservative in desiccated coconut, you can process fresh coconut in a food processor.
Pure maple syrup may be used as an alternative to honey.

Slices
All slices are made by pressing mixture into a rectangular oven-proof dish approximately 27 cm. by 16 cm. The cooked slab should be cut into squares while hot. Also, to prevent sticking, run a knife around the sides of the dish while hot. Remove slices when cool. Soak dish before washing.

Muesli Slice
½ cup flour
1½ cups oats

1 cup coconut or sesame seeds
½ cup ground nuts
1½ cups dried fruit
1 tablesp. honey
1 tablesp. coconut oil
1 cup water

1. Mix all ingredients together.
2. Add extra water if necessary until the mixture has a stiff, moist consistency.
3. Spread mixture into a rectangular oven-proof dish. (27 cm. by 16 cm.)
4. Bake 20 minutes in a moderate oven.
5. Remove from oven and cut into slices, but don't remove slices from dish until cool.

Oatmeal Slice

½ cup flour
1½ cups oats
1 cup coconut or sesame seeds
½ cup ground nuts/ sunflower seeds
1 tablespoons honey
1 tablesp. coconut oil
½ teasp. ginger
1 teasp. cinnamon
1 cup water

1. Mix all ingredients together.
2. Add enough water to make a moist but stiff consistency.
3. Spread mixture into a rectangular oven-proof dish. (27 cm. by 16 cm.)
4. Bake 20 minutes in moderate oven.
5. Cut into squares while hot and remove slices when cold.

This can be used as a base for fruit tarts.

Gluten-free slice

1 cup brown rice flour
1 cup ground nuts
1 cup coconut or sesame seeds

½ cup chopped nuts or sunflower seeds
1½ cups dried fruit
1 tablesp. honey
1 tablesp. coconut oil
½ cup water

1. Mix all ingredients together.
2. Add extra water if necessary until the mixture has a stiff, moist consistency.
3. Spread mixture into a rectangular oven-proof dish.
4. Bake 20 minutes in a moderate oven.
5. Remove from oven and cut into slices, but don't remove slices from dish until cool.

Carrot Slice

2 - 3 medium carrots (140 g.)
½ cup walnuts (chopped)
½ cup dates, raisins or sultanas
1 cups oats
1 cup flour
2 tablesp. honey
1 dessertsp. olive oil or coconut oil
50 ml. water (just under ¼ cup)

1. Grate carrots or use in food processor.
2. Mix all ingredients together except for water.
3. Add just enough water to make a sticky consistency.
4. Press into rectangular oven-proof dish.
5. Bake 20 minutes in a moderate.
6. Cut into squares while hot. Remove when cold.

COOKIES AND TRUFFLES
Carob Cookies

1 cup oats
1 cup flour
1 cup coconut or sesame seeds
1 cup almond or sunflower seeds, ground
1 tablesp. carob powder

2 tablesp. honey
1 tablesp. coconut oil
100 ml. water

1. Mix all ingredients together, water last. Add enough water to make a firm mixture.
2. Place in spoonfuls on a tray and flatten with a fork.
3. Bake moderate oven 5 minutes. Loosen the cookies form tray as soon as they come out of the oven.

For a different flavour, carob powder can be substituted with cinnamon, mixed spice or ginger.

Banana Date Cookies
1- 2 ripe bananas
½ cup raisins
1 cup almonds, ground
1 cup rolled oats

1. Grind nuts.
2. Mash one ripe banana.
3. Mix all ingredients with the mashed banana so that mixture sticks together.
4. Add more mashed banana if necessary.
5. Roll into balls and flatten with a fork on a baking tray.
6. Bake at 180 degrees C for 20 minutes. Remove from tray while hot.

Apple and Date Cookies
1 cup almonds, ground
1 cup apple puree, stewed with honey
1 cup oats
½ cup dates
1 tablesp. boiling water

1. Chop dates and stand in a bowl with the boiling water for 5 minutes.
2. Combine all dry ingredients.
3. Drain dates. Combine dates and stewed apple puree with dry ingredients.
4. Form balls and flatten with a fork on a baking tray.
5. Bake at 180 degrees C for 20 minutes. Remove from tray while hot.

Gingerbread Cookies

1½ cups flour
½ teasp. baking powder
3 tablesp. cold-pressed olive oil
2 tablesp. honey
½ teasp. ginger
1 teasp. cinnamon

1. Mix all ingredients together.
2. Knead.
3. Chill.
4. Roll out on floured board and cut cookie shapes.
5. Bake in a moderate oven for 7 minutes.

Truffles

2 cups oats
1 dessertsp. carob powder
1 dessertsp. honey or pure maple syrup
1 cup coconut or sesame seeds
½ cup sultanas
½ cup ground almonds
2 tablesp. coconut oil

1. Place all ingredients in the food processor. Blend.
2. Form balls. Alternatively, spoon into patti-pans.
3. Chill.

Oats may be used raw, or pre-baked on a tray in the oven for a few minutes.

Fruit Balls

½ cup of each of the following:
dates, sultanas, dried apricots, nuts
1 cup coconut or oats
2 tablesp. fresh orange juice.

1. Soak fruit in boiling water first, to soften, then drain.
2. Place all ingredients in the food processor. Blend nuts first, then add other ingredients.
3. Form into balls.

4. Chill.
Oats may be used raw, or pre-baked on a tray in the oven for a few minutes.

DESSERTS AND AFTERNOON TEAS

Nut Pastry
½ cup wholemeal flour
½ cup buckwheat flour
½ cup barley or millet flour
½ cup ground almonds or cashews
½ cup water
1 dessertsp. cold-pressed olive oil

1. Grind nuts in food processor until fine.
2. Add flours and olive oil.
3. Add enough water while blending to make a firm dough.
4. Chill and roll out.

This recipe will also work with all wheat-free flours.

Custard
2 tablesp. brown rice flour or cornflour
2 cups cold water, or 1 cup water plus 1 cup non-homogenised goat milk
1 tablesp. honey
1 egg

Method 1
1. Place all ingredients in a blender and blend.
2. Transfer mixture to a saucepan and stir until boiling. Add natural vanilla essence.

Method 2
1. Whisk the flour and rice flour with the cold water, in a saucepan.
2. Add egg and honey and continue to whisk over the heat, until honey melts.
3. Change to wooden spoon and stir until mixture comes to the boil.
4. Add few drops of natural vanilla essence.
5. Sprinkle with sesame seeds or granola. Served cold, for mixing with apricot kernels.

Add cooked rice for rice custard.

Fruit Pies

quantity of stewed fruit sweetened with fruit concentrate or honey
quantity of 'Nut Pastry'.
1. Prepare pastry and roll out pie shell.
2. Place in an oven-proof dish and bake for about 5 minutes.
3. Pour filling into shell.
4. Place a layer of pastry on top and bake in moderate oven for about 25 minutes.

Lemon Pie

quantity of 'Nut Pastry'
½ cup almonds
2 tablesp. honey
1 tablesp. lemon juice
small piece lemon rind
3 teaspoons cornflour or rice flour
1 cup water
1 egg

1. Prepare pastry. Roll out and make a pie shell. Bake the pie shell 10 minutes.
2. Place cornflour, lemon juice, honey, and egg in cold water in saucepan. Whisk while bringing to the boil.
3. In food processor, process almonds until very fine. Stir into custard.
4. Pour mixture into baked pastry shell.

Pumpkin Pie

quantity 'Nut Pastry'
2 cups cooked, mashed pumpkin
2 eggs
2 tablesp. honey
1 teasp. cinnamon
½ teasp. ginger
½ teasp. spice
1 cup rice milk or non-homogenised goat milk

1. Prepare pastry and roll out pie crust. Bake 10 minutes.
2. Combine all ingredients and mix well.
3. Pour into pie crust and bake moderate oven for 40 minutes.

Frozen Fruit Sorbet
(A good summer afternoon snack for children)
Freeze pieces of fruit – e.g. berries, mango, bananas, and put through a centrifuge juicer.

Carrot Cake
150 g. carrots (approx. 3 medium carrots)
½ cup brazil nuts or walnuts
3 eggs
3 tablesp. cold-pressed olive oil
1 cup plain wholemeal flour
1 teasp. cinnamon
¼ teasp. nutmeg
1 cup coconut or oat bran
3 tablesp. honey
1 tablesp. water

1. Process nuts and carrots in food processor, (or chop and grate by hand if you prefer).
2. Transfer to a bowl. Stir in eggs, then all other ingredients except water.
3. Add as much water as you need to get a good 'dropping' consistency, (not a 'pouring' consistency).
4. Bake in a moderate oven for about 40 minutes.

This cake contains no rising agent except for eggs and therefore makes a heavy cake.

Apple and Raisin Cake
2 cups diced apple
1½ cups flour
2 eggs (medium or large)
1 cup chopped raisins or sultanas
1 teasp. cinnamon
½ teasp. ground cloves
½ teasp. grated nutmeg
2 tablesp. honey
2 tablesp. cold-pressed olive oil
60 g. walnuts, pecans or almonds

1. Mix apples and honey.
2. Add beaten eggs raisins and nuts.
3. Add oil and sifted dry ingredients.
4. Grease the sides of a ring tin with olive oil and line the base with baking paper.
5. Bake in moderate oven 50 minutes.

This cake contains no rising agent except for eggs, and therefore makes a heavier cake. Delicious served warm.

Hot Fruit Salad

Eat fruit on and empty stomach, e.g. for mid-afternoon snack,(not following a meal).

4 cups of fresh fruit, chopped in chunky pieces
1 tablesp. honey
½ cup orange juice
½ cup dried fruit, soaked in cup orange juice

1. Place dried fruit in saucepan and bring dried fruit to boil and simmer 1 minute.
2. Prepare fresh fruit. Add fresh fruit to dried fruit and orange sauce.
3. Serve.

Fresh fruit should be hot but not cooked. May be spiced with ginger.
Serve as a single dish for afternoon tea. (Eat fruit on an empty stomach.)

Sago Delight

½ cup sago
2 tablesp. honey
1 cup tinned berries or apricots

1. Boil sago with 1½ cups of liquid, (water plus juice from fruit), until soft and light.
2. Add fruit and honey.
3. Stir 1 minute over heat.
4. Cool and chill.

Apricot Delight

quantity of 'Nut Pastry'
1 tablesp. arrowroot

2 cups apricot nectar
juice of 1 orange
250 g. dried apricots
¼ teasp. cinnamon
1 tablesp. honey

1. Prepare pastry and line a pie dish. Bake 10 minutes.
2. Whisk together in a saucepan, apricot nectar, orange juice and arrowroot. Add honey. Stir until it comes to the boil.
3. Add cinnamon and dried apricots.
4. Pour into pastry shell and chill.

Fruit Jelly
1 teasp. agar agar powder
1 cup fruit juice e.g. grape juice
450 g. fruit

1. Place fruit in the bottom of an oven-proof dish.
2. Whisk the agar agar powder together with juice, in a saucepan over heat.
3. Continue to stir until boiling.
4. Pour hot jelly over fruit. Cool and refrigerate.

Fruit Crumble
4 cups of stewed fruit
Topping:
1 tablesp. rolled oats (chopped finely in food processor)
1 tablesp. sesame seeds
½ teasp. cinnamon
1 tablesp. coconut or oatbran
1 tablesp. flour
1 tablesp. fruit juice concentrate or honey
1 teasp. olive oil
1. Place stewed fruit in casserole dish.
2. Mix topping ingredients together and sprinkle over stewed fruit. Bake 15-20 minutes.

Creamed Rice with Dates
3 cups cooked brown rice
2 cups rice milk

½ cup dates
1. Blend dates with rice milk.
2. Pour over rice and warm through.

Cakes

The following recipes contain baking powder, which may reduce the efficiency of the digestive system and interfere with the absorption of iron. Recipes in this section should therefore be reserved for special occasions. The non-aluminium baking powder available from health shops is best. Also remember that wheat flour does not have to be used. Spelt flour, millet flour and buckwheat flour can all be used.

Porridge Cake

1 cup flour
1 teasp. baking powder
1½ cups oats
3 tablesp. honey
½ teasp. each ginger and mixed spice
2 tablesp. cold-pressed olive oil
1 cup water

1. Mix all ingredients together. The consistency should be a moist and sticky.
2. Line the bottom of the tin with baking paper. Pour in mixture.
3. Bake in a loaf tin at 180 degrees C for about 40 minutes.

Apple Cake

1 cup flour
1 teasp. baking powder
1½ cups oats
3 tablesp. honey
½ teasp. each ginger and cinnamon
3 tablsp. cold pressed oil
2 cups dried apples roughly chopped
2 cups water

1. Boil dried apples with water for 5 minutes.
2. Mix all ingredients together except for apples.
3. Drain apples and stir into mixture.
4. Add a little liquid from the saucepan. Use as much liquid as necessary to

make a moist, sticky 'dropping' consistency.
5. Bake in a moderate oven 40 minutes.
Fresh apples may be used in place of dried apples for a consistency that is less chewy. Prepare 2 large apples and cook for 2 minutes in a little honey or fruit juice concentrate.

Fruit Cake
2 cups flour
1 teasp. baking powder
2 eggs
3 cups dried fruit
2 teasp. spice
1 cup water
2 tablesp. fruit juice concentrate
1 tablesp. honey
3 tablesp. cold-pressed olive oil

1. Boil fruit, water, fruit juice concentrate and honey. Simmer and cool.
2. Stir in beaten eggs and flour.
3. Stir in spice, baking powder and cold-pressed oil. If mixture is too stiff add a little water.
4. Bake 1 hour in a moderate oven.

Eggless Fruit Cake
1 cup dried fruit
2 cups flour
1 teasp. baking powder
2 tablesp. honey
1½ cups cold fruit tea or green tea (tea bag)

1. Soak fruit in tea overnight.
2. Stir in all other ingredients into the soaked fruit and liquid.
3. Bake moderate oven 1 hour.

Coconut Fruit Cake
2 cups dried fruit
1½ cups apple juice
75 g. walnuts

1½ cups coconut or oat bran
1½ cups flour
2 teasp. baking powder

1. Soak dried fruit in apple juice 2 hours.
2. Add other ingredients.
3. Bake 1 hour 170 degrees C.

Sultana Muffins
1 cup flour
1 cup baking flour
1 cup coconut or oat bran
1 cup sultanas
½ cup organic natural yoghurt
½ cup water
1 tablesp. honey

1. Mix all ingredients together.
2. Place mixture into muffin tins.
3. Bake at 180 degrees for 20 minutes.
Natural yoghurt may be replaced with water or fruit juice.

Apple Muffins
1 cup flour
1 teasp. baking flour
1 cup coconut or oat bran
1 cup chopped raw apple
½ cup organic natural yoghurt
½ cup water
1 tablesp. honey

1. Mix all ingredients together.
2. Place mixture into muffin tins.
3. Bake at 180 degrees for about 20 minutes.
Substitute other fruits – e.g. chopped banana as desired.
Water may be used in place of natural yoghurt

Dried Fruit Muffins

1 cup dried fruit
½ cup fruit juice
1 cup flour
1 teasp. baking powder
1 egg
¼ cup water
2 tablesp. coconut oil
1 tablesp. honey

1. Soak dried fruit in fruit juice for at least an hour.
2. Mix all ingredients together, stirring in water last. Add gradually, until mixture is the right consistency.
3. Place mixture into muffin tins.
4. Bake at 180 degrees for 15 minutes.

Dates, sultanas, raisins, dried apple, dried apricots are all suitable. Add spices if desired.

Fresh Fruit Muffins

½ cup fresh fruit, chopped
½ cup fruit juice
1 cup flour
1 teasp. baking powder
1 egg
1 tablesp. coconut oil
1 tablesp. honey

1. Mix all ingredients together, stirring in fruit last.
2. Place mixture in muffin tins.
3. Bake at 180 degrees for 15-20 minutes.

Fresh berries, fresh apple and banana are all suitable.

Carob Muffins

1 cup flour
1 teasp. baking powder
1 tablesp. carob powder
2 tablesp. honey
1 egg

½ cup organic natural yoghurt

1. Mix all ingredients together.
2. Place mixture in muffin tin.
3. Bake at 180 degrees for 15 minutes.
Water may be used in place of natural yoghurt.

13. BREAD

Wholemeal Bread
Mix the following ingredients together:
2½ cups wholemeal spelt flour
2½ cups white spelt flour
½ cup gluten flour
1 cup barley or millet flour
1 tablesp. yeast

Mix the following together in a jug:
600 ml. hot water (400 ml. boiling water, 200 ml. cool water)
1 tablesp. honey
2 tablesp. tahini or cold-pressed olive oil
½ teasp. Celtic salt

1. Add the wet ingredients in the jug to the dry ingredients. Mix. Add more water or flour if needed so that a firm, moist dough is achieved.
2. Cover with plastic wrap and a towel. Allow to rise 20-30 minutes.
3. Turn onto a floured board and knead approximately 10 minutes. The longer you knead the softer the bread will be.
4. Divide in half and shape each half into a ball and place onto a floured baking tray. (Use bread tins in you prefer.)
5. Let rise approximately 15-20 minutes.
6. Place in a pre-heated oven at 180 degrees for 10 minutes then reduce to 150 degrees for another 30 minutes.

14. THERMOMIX RECIPES
Thermomix is a time-saving food processing machine that chops, grates, stirs and cooks. Most of the recipes in this book can be made with Thermomix. However, the following recipes give specific instructions for Thermomix.

Coleslaw
100 g. carrots
250 g. red cabbage
1 stick celery
¼ salad onion or chopped chives
½ cup walnut pieces
1 tablesp. lemon juice
1 teasp. honey

Place all ingredients in bowl except for nuts. Chop for 15-18 seconds on speed 3 with aid of spatula. Stir in nuts on speed 1.

Beetroot salad
1 raw beetroot
1 carrot
1 stick celery
¼ red salad onion or some chopped chives
fresh parsley
½ teasp. Celtic salt
1 dessertsp. lemon juice
1 teasp. honey

Place all ingredients in bowl. Chop for 20 seconds on speed 3.

Minestrone
400 g. red kidney beans, (cooked)
400 g. tomatoes
1 clove garlic
1 piece capsicum
1 stick celery
1 carrot
basil and oregano
1 dessertsp. olive oil
1 teasp. Celtic salt, or 1 vegetable stock cube
500 ml. water

Drop onion and garlic on rotating blades. Chop on speed 4 for 5 seconds. Add oil. Saute 2 minutes at 100 degrees on speed 1. Add celery, (with leaves), carrot, capsicum, herbs, tomatoes and half of the cooked beans. Pulverise 30 seconds on speed 6. Add water and salt and the rest of the beans. Cook for 20 minutes, speed 1.

Chick Pea Soup
2 cups chick peas, soaked and rinsed
900 ml water
100 g. each potato, pumpkin, sweet potato
1 medium carrot
1 stick celery
1 piece capsicum
1 onion
1 teasp. cumin
1 teasp. turmeric
1 teasp. coriander

Chop vegetables on speed 4 for 15 seconds. Add water and pulverise on speed 9 for 10 seconds. Add chick peas and cook at 100 degrees, speed 2 for 30 minutes.

Thick Red Lentils
2 cups red lentils, soaked and rinsed
400 g. tin tomatoes
550 ml. water
1 onion
2 teasp. Celtic salt
1 teasp. dried herbs – basil and oregano, or 1 teasp. curry powder

Drop onion on chopping blades, speed 8. Add tomatoes, water and herbs or spices. Blend on speed 9 for 10 seconds. Add lentils. Cook for 30 minutes at 100 degrees, speed 2. Add Celtic salt and stir on speed 2 for 10 seconds.

Savoury Cashew Spread
200 g. raw cashews
1 cup water
3 heaped teasp. arrowroot or cornflour
1 teasp. Celtic salt
¼ teasp. sweet paprika
1 teasp. onion powder

Place the water and arrowroot in the bowl. Blend on speed 9. Cook for 6 minutes at 100 degrees, speed 2. Transfer this mixture into a crockery bowl and allow to cool. Place nuts, Celtic salt and spices in bowl and grind on Speed 9. Add cooled arrowroot paste to the bowl. Stir with spatula. Blend on speed 9 for 10 seconds. Stir with spatula and blend again for another 10 seconds.

Nut Burgers

1 onion
½ teasp. dried herbs
2 slices good bread
1 dessertsp. savoury yeast flakes, or ½ stock cube
1 dessertsp kelp sauce or tamari
½ small zucchini (100 g.) or 1 stick celery
1½ cups sunflower seeds or nuts
¼ cup water

Grind nuts or sunflower seeds for 10 seconds on speed 8. Add onion, zucchini and bread and chop on speed 4. Add water, herbs and yeast flakes and blend on speed 6 for 15 seconds. Stir with spatula and blend again for 10 seconds. Make patties or burgers by spooning out mixture into a hot pan greased with olive oil. Turn patties 3 times. To get the last of the mixture off the blades and out of the bowl, run the machine on speed 6 for a few seconds and scrape down sides with spatula.

Custard

Piece of lemon rind
1 tablesp. honey
2 eggs
375 ml. water
375 ml. non-homogenised goat milk
3 tablesp. brown rice flour

Drop lemon rind on to rotating blades, speed 9 for 5 seconds. Scrape down with spatula. Add all other ingredients. Blend on speed 9 for 20 seconds. Cook on speed 4 for 6 minutes at 80 degrees.

Agar Fruit Jelly
500 ml. fruit juice
20 g. agar agar flakes, or 1 tsp. powder
450 g. berries or fresh fruit of your choice

Place fruit on the bottom of a large bowl. Place juice and agar agar into the bowl and mix for 10 seconds on speed 9. Bring the mixture to the boil by cooking for 4 minutes at 100 degrees on speed 4. Allow to cool for a couple of minutes, then slowly pour the jelly over the fruits. Allow to set for approximately 1–2 hours at room temperature.

Taiwanese Porridge
20 g. brown rice
40 g. quinoa
20 g. rolled oats
20 g. nuts
20 g. sesame/ sunflower seeds
1 litre water
½ teasp. Celtic salt
Maple syrup

Place dry ingredients in the bowl and mill for 1 minute on speed 8. Add water and cook for 15 minutes at 100 degrees on speed 4. Add salt and mix for a further 20 seconds on speed 6. Serve with maple syrup.

CONTACTS AND ADDITIONAL RESOURCES

For further information on availability of products and ingredients visit
www.beaconmedia.com.au

The Healthy Food Guide – for children and their parents
This is a series of lessons in healthy eating, for primary-age children.
www.beaconmedia.com.au

Living Valley Springs Health Retreat
For live-in cleanse therapy
www.lvs.com.au

Thermomix
www.thermomix.com.au

To contact the author please email:
info@beaconmedia.com.au

INDEX

Acid-alkaline balance 31
Additives 41, 47, 57, 60, 72, 108
Allergies 10, 16, 21, 26, 29, 31, 57, 73, 112
Amalgam fillings 62, 63, 82
Antibiotics 19, 20, 21, 51, 53, 63, 102, 110
Antioxidants 14, 23, 28, 59, 63, 78, 90, 83, 87-89, 94, 98, 99
Apricot kernels 54, 72, 77, 185
Artificial colourings and flavourings 9, 26
Aspartame 28

Baking powder 25, 37, 74
Betacarotene 69, 76, 80, 89
Blood pressure 29, 30
Bovine cartilage 86
Bread 16, 20, 24, 25, 26, 41, 42, 46, 74, 98, 101, 119, 120, 126, 132, 134, 136, 138, 152, 158, 162, 164-167, 172, 173, 175, 180, 183, 189, 192
Budget 44
Butter 17, 29, 40, 44

Caffeine 29, 73, 74, 102
Cakes 25, 41, 42, 44, 100, 128, 176, 178, 180
Calcium 16, 21, 22, 30, 35, 37, 48, 87, 90, 95, 102-103
Cancer 10, 14, 16, 18, 19, 21, 24, 25-28, 35-37, 41, 48, 51-53, 57-64, 67-96, 107
Candida 16, 22, 26, 63
Canola oil 17, 40
Carbohydrates 15, 23, 74, 98, 100
Carcinogenic 15, 17, 18, 40, 74, 75
Cheese 22, 25, 41, 42, 44, 130, 135, 139, 153, 159, 160, 162, 180
Chelation therapy 88, 95, 96, 103
Chicken 20, 22, 29
Children 9, 10, 11, 14, 17, 20, 22, 23, 26, 31, 36, 40, 41, 42, 48, 53, 64, 88, 91, 99, 111
China Project, the 58, 59, 65
Chocolate 27, 29, 30, 33
Coffee 18, 30, 31, 72, 74, 77, 99, 103
Cruciferous vegetables 15, 69
Dairy 17, 21, 22, 32, 35, 40, 42, 44, 47, 58, 71, 73, 81, 94, 99, 102-103, 112
Depression 18, 25, 31, 42, 52, 57
Diabetes 18, 23, 89, 93, 99, 100, 107
Eggs 17, 20, 21, 22, 23, 25, 32, 36, 37, 47, 48, 53, 59, 62, 63, 71, 81, 89, 99, 122, 150, 166, 175, 186, 187, 192

Enzymes 15, 25, 54, 59, 62, 70-72, 87, 90, 97
Essiac tea 77, 79
Essential fatty acids 18, 36

Fat 16, 17, 18, 19, 21, 22, 25, 26, 28, 32, 36, 45, 48, 51, 57, 58, 59, 61, 62, 63, 72, 72, 94, 96, 98, 100, 102-103, 106, 112
Fatigue 25, 28, 51, 53, 57, 97
Fibre 16, 58, 70, 74, 100
Fish 18, 19, 36, 37, 59
Fish oil 18, 19, 36, 37, 48, 59, 71, 103
Flaxseed 18
Food additives 10, 11, 26, 32, 41, 57, 73
Free radicals 14, 63, 83, 87, 89
Fruit 11, 14-17, 22, 23, 25, 30, 32, 35, 36, 39, 40, 42, 44, 46, 54, 59, 68, 69, 70, 71, 75-78, 85, 86, 89-90, 98-99, 102, 107, 112, 121, 125, 126, 131-133, 135-137, 139, 180, 181, 184-188, 192, 193,196

Gerson, Max 25, 37, 67, 68, 79, 81, 85, 87
Grains 11, 14, 15, 16, 21, 23, 32, 35, 36, 37, 68, 76, 89, 124, 129, 141, 168
Grape seed 15, 28, 78, 80, 87
Green barley 32, 77, 79, 90

Heart disease 14, 17, 18, 22, 30, 35, 36, 42, 58, 89, 93, 94, 96, 107, 112
Herbs 15, 48, 63, 68, 71, 80, 85, 110, 127, 128, 138, 140, 153-158, 162, 167, 168, 172-174, 180, 190-191
Homogenisation 22
Honey 23, 25, 36, 77, 97, 101, 132, 135, 137, 139, 146, 148, 154, 180-192
Hormonal balance 32, 103

Iron 15, 16, 21, 25, 30, 37, 41, 48, 74, 83, 87, 89-90, 98
Juicing 69, 70, 81, 89

Krebs, Dr. Ernst 72

Lead 19, 23, 30, 62, 68, 85, 88, 93-95
Lentils 22, 25, 35, 36, 37, 40, 42, 44, 45, 46, 53, 71, 76, 98, 101, 122, 126, 127, 129, 136, 146, 147, 153, 155, 157-159, 163, 171, 191
Leucosis 20
Lymphoma 27, 51, 52, 53

Magnesium 29, 30, 48, 83, 87, 102, 103
Margarine 17, 25, 40, 41, 71, 74, 94
Meat 17, 19, 20, 21, 22, 35, 37, 40-47, 58, 59, 71, 73, 75, 81, 94, 99, 101, 106-111
Mercury 17-19, 36, 37, 48, 62, 71, 82, 103

Microwave ovens 63, 75, 76
Milk substitutes 40
Minerals 9, 14, 15, 16, 21, 23, 24, 36, 37, 48, 59, 68, 77, 81, 82, 83, 85-87, 90, 93, 94, 98, 100, 103

Nuts 11, 14, 16, 17, 19, 21, 25, 35, 36, 37, 41, 44, 46, 48, 76, 77, 85, 94, 95, 96, 98-100, 102, 121, 122, 128-133, 138, 146, 149-151, 160, 162, 167, 170, 180-187, 190, 193

Oil 15, 17-19, 25, 32, 36, 37, 40, 41, 44, 48, 63, 75, 89, 100, 103
Olive oil 18, 19, 25, 32, 37, 41, 44, 48, 63, 89, 122, 123, 133, 139, 142-175, 179, 184-186, 190, 192
Omega-3, omega-6 18, 19, 36, 77
Osteoporosis 22, 23, 48, 58, 89, 93, 102-103, 107

Parasites 63
Peanut butter 17
Peanuts 17
Polysaccharides 15, 80, 89-90
Pork 17
Potassium 16, 24, 25, 29, 83, 87, 90, 102
Preservatives 9, 20, 26, 28, 29, 47, 57, 73
Price, Weston 59
Protein 16, 17, 19, 21, 22, 35, 36, 37, 47, 48, 57, 58, 59, 68, 70, 72, 73, 86, 90, 98, 100, 102, 108

Salmonella 19, 35
Salt 11, 16, 24, 26, 32, 42, 57, 73, 77
Seeds 11, 14, 16, 17, 18, 19, 21, 32, 36, 37, 41, 44, 48, 71, 72, 76, 78, 87, 89, 98, 99, 121, 122, 126, 129-131, 133, 136, 238-139, 144-147, 150-152, 154, 156-161, 164, 167-168, 180-182, 184-185, 192, 193
Selenium 83
Sodium 22, 24, 25, 60, 83, 98
Spices 26, 125, 155, 156, 190
Spirulina 32, 37, 77, 78, 80, 89, 90
Stroke 89, 92
Sugar 10, 11, 16, 23, 24, 25, 28 30, 32, 36, 40, 42, 48, 57, 63, 71, 73, 74, 77, 86, 96, 99, 108, 121, 123, 124
Supplements 40, 48, 52, 53, 54, 59, 72, 77, 80, 81, 85, 86, 88, 90

Tahini 17, 41, 48, 126, 131-132, 134, 161, 163-164, 166, 169, 189
Tea 10, 14, 30, 31, 32, 44, 73, 77, 79-80, 82, 87, 98-99, 103, 135
Toxic, toxins 9, 10, 18, 19, 24, 27, 29, 30, 40, 54, 57, 59, 60, 61, 62, 64, 65, 68, 71, 72-76, 81-82, 88-91, 93-94, 98, 102, 112-113

Vegetables 11, 14, 15, 16, 17, 19, 21, 22, 23, 24, 25, 30, 32, 35, 36, 37, 40, 42, 43, 44, 46, 53, 59, 68, 69, 70, 71, 75, 76, 79, 80, 82, 89-90, 97-99, 101-102, 112, 121, 124, 128-129, 140-141, 143-144, 146, 149, 150-156, 158, 160-161, 163, 165, 169, 174, 178-179, 191
Viruses 9, 15, 19, 106, 112
Vitamins 9, 14, 15, 16, 17, 23, 24, 29, 36, 37, 48, 59, 72, 85, 88, 90, 94, 100, 103
Vitamin B12 21, 37, 41, 48
Vitamin B17 16, 54, 71, 72, 77
Vitamin C 16, 21, 37, 73, 78, 87-89
Vitamin E 18, 28, 37, 83, 89-90

Water 13, 14, 25, 30, 31, 33, 44, 45, 59, 67, 68, 71, 77, 78, 79-82, 94, 98-99, 102, 106
Weight loss 96-97, 100
Wheat 15, 16, 70, 71,
Wheat grass 70, 71
Whole grains 15, 16, 21, 23, 35, 36, 37, 76, 89

Yeast 22, 26, 57, 63, 74, 130, 167, 189, 192
Yoghurt 22, 37, 40, 53, 123, 139, 145-146, 152, 187-189, 198

Zinc 73, 87, 90, 102

Change your life...

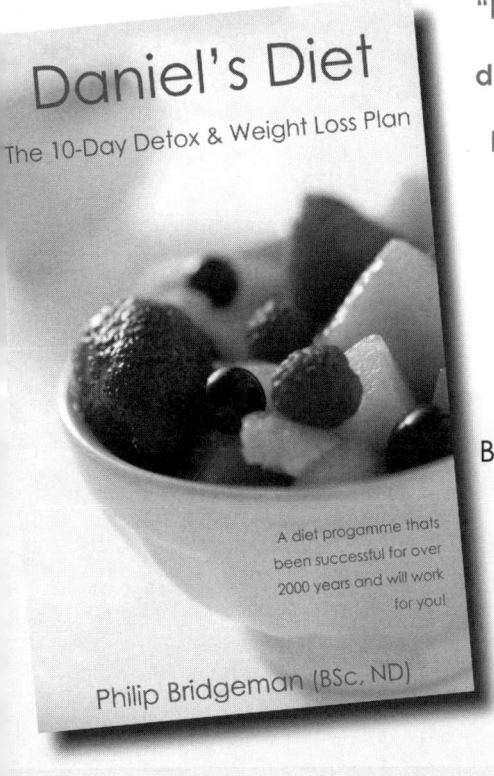

Daniel's Diet
The 10-Day Detox & Weight Loss Plan

A diet progamme thats been successful for over 2000 years and will work for you!

Philip Bridgeman (BSc, ND)

"Daniel's Diet is not just another diet book. This book is different. It's God's own diet drawn from His word."

Dr Cecile Lombard MD

Based on Daniel's diet from the book of Daniel—Naturopath & Nutritionist Philip Bridgeman has devised a 10-day detox and weight loss plan based on the scriptures, that actually works!

Daniel's Diet bridges the 2500-year gap between then and now.

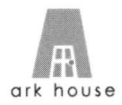

Available in all good bookstores throughout Australia and New Zealand or go to www.arkhousepress.com

ark house

Subscribe...

to Australia and New Zealand's leading Christian magazine.

- health
- parenting
- real stories
- leadership
- recipes
- + MORE

For over 50 years, Christian Woman has been inspiring, challenging and encouraging women of all ages in their daily life.

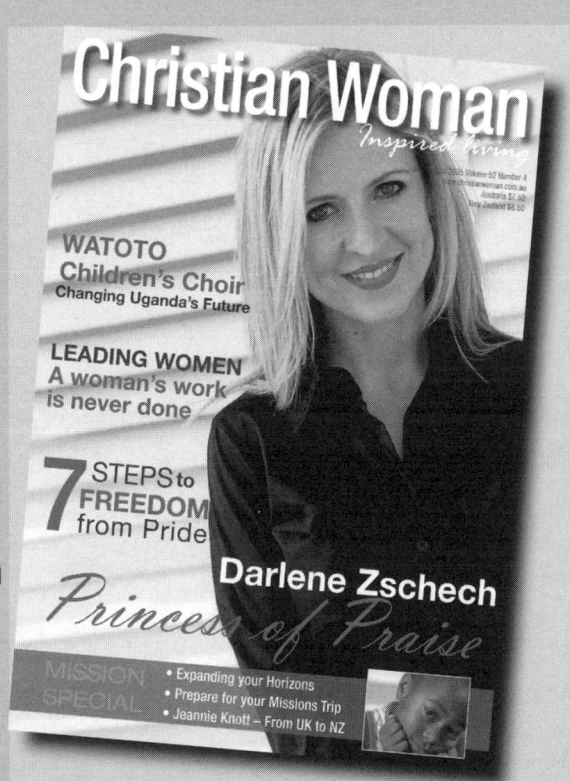

Christian Woman
Inspired living

www.christianwoman.com.au